# Veterinary Medical School Admission Requirements

# Veterinary Medical School Admission Requirements

**2014 EDITION FOR 2015 MATRICULATION**

ASSOCIATION OF AMERICAN VETERINARY MEDICAL COLLEGES

PURDUE UNIVERSITY PRESS | WEST LAFAYETTE, INDIANA

Compiled by the Association of American Veterinary Medical Colleges;
Tony Wynne, Editor, Director of Admissions and Recruitment Affairs

Cover photograph courtesy of Auburn University
Back cover photographs courtesy of:
1. North Carolina State University
2. University of California, Davis

Paperback ISBN: 978-155753-679-2
ePub ISBN: 978-1-61249-320-6
ePDF ISBN: 978-1-61249-319-0
ISSN: 1089-6465

# APRIL 15TH ACCEPTANCE DEADLINE POLICY

In order to grant member schools enough time to complete their admissions processes and for applicants to make informed admissions decisions, schools will not require applicants to decide upon admissions offers, scholarships, and financial aid until April 15. To ensure applicant awareness of this policy, the schools will attach the policy to all admissions offer letters. If April 15 falls upon a weekend, the date will be shifted to the next Monday. This policy does not apply to the following schools: International Schools; Tuskegee University.

**Approved by the AAVMC Board of Directors**
July 17, 2011

# CONTENTS

# FOREWORD

The profession of veterinary medicine plays a critical role in the health and wellbeing of our rapidly changing world. Spanning many different dimensions of animal and human health, veterinary medicine offers an array of exciting, enriching, and fulfilling career choices. Getting started and making sense of all the options and requirements can seem challenging, but you'll find this publication a helpful resource.

All of the veterinary colleges and schools highlighted in this publication are accredited by the American Veterinary Medical Association (AVMA) or are engaged in the accreditation process. This book will help you understand and consider important factors like cost, financial aid, potential debt, special programs, standardized tests, the AAVMC Veterinary Medical College Application Service (VM-CAS), and the various colleges' and schools' residency admissions requirements.

> Perhaps no other medical career provides such a broad base of biomedical training and leads to so many different areas of opportunity.

Like other health professions, the pursuit and achievement of a veterinary medical education represents a considerable investment of time, effort and financial resources. Cost-saving strategies include focusing on in-state veterinary medical schools or states that offer in-state tuition as part of special agreements with neighboring states. Other strategies include focusing on areas of greatest need, such as rural veterinary practice where loan repayment options might be available.

Our profession offers many opportunities beyond the time-honored practice of providing clinical care in general practice. Earning professional certification can lead to specialty practice in surgery, internal medicine, ophthalmology, and many other areas. Rewarding public health careers are available with national and international groups like the Centers for Disease Control (CDC), the World Health Organization (WHO), and other groups. You can prepare yourself for scientific and administrative careers with pharmaceutical, nutrition and biomedical health corporations, or work in state and federal government. Conducting graduate work to complement your professional degree can lead to faculty positions in higher education.

More information can be found on individual college and school websites or on the AAVMC website at www.aavmc.org. Prospective students also can contact the appropriate admissions office at each school or the VMCAS Student and Advisor Hotline, either by e-mail (vmcasinfo@vmcas.org) or by calling VMCAS at (617) 612-2884.

We congratulate you for your decision to pursue a career in veterinary medicine. Perhaps no other medical career provides such a broad base of biomedical training and leads to so many different areas of opportunity. In my own case, a veterinary medical education has led me to service as an officer in the United States Air Force, work in a mixed animal practice, in public health as an official with the U.S. Centers for Disease Control and Prevention, and now, as executive director of the AAVMC.

All of us at the AAVMC wish you luck and success as you prepare yourself for service in this extraordinary and rewarding profession.

**Dr. Andrew Maccabe**
AAVMC Executive Director

# ABOUT THE AAVMC

The Association of American Veterinary Medical Colleges (AAVMC) is a non-profit membership organization working to protect and improve the health and welfare of animals, people, and the environment by advancing academic veterinary medicine. The association was founded in 1966 by the deans of the then-existing eighteen colleges of veterinary medicine in the United States and three in Canada. During the 1970s and 1980s, AAVMC's membership expanded to include departments of veterinary science in colleges of agriculture, and in the 1990s to include divisions or departments of comparative medicine. In 2008, AAVMC began accepting non-accredited colleges and schools of veterinary medicine as affiliate members.

Today, AAVMC provides leadership for an academic veterinary medical community that includes all thirty colleges of veterinary medicine in the United States; nine departments of veterinary science; eight departments of comparative medicine; all five veterinary medical colleges in Canada; thirteen accredited colleges of veterinary medicine in Australia, Grenada, Ireland, Mexico, the Netherlands, New Zealand, St. Kitts, the United Kingdom, and six affiliate members.

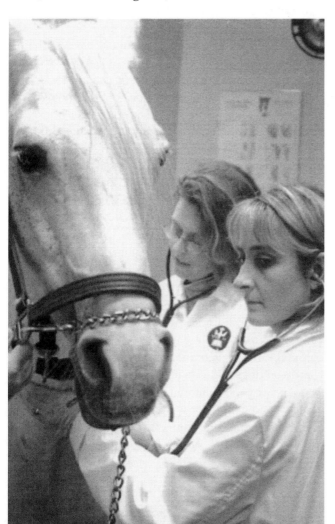

## MISSION

AAVMC provides leadership for and promotes excellence in academic veterinary medicine to prepare the veterinary workforce with the scientific knowledge and skills required to meet societal needs through the protection of animal health, the relief of animal suffering, the conservation of animal resources, the promotion of public health, and the advancement of medical knowledge.

AAVMC pursues its mission by providing leadership in:
- Advocating on behalf of academic veterinary medicine;
- Serving as a catalyst and convener on issues of importance to academic veterinary medicine;
- Providing information, knowledge, and solutions to support members' work;
- Facilitating enrollment in veterinary medical schools and colleges; and
- Building global partnerships and coalitions to advance our collective goals.

## STRATEGIC GOALS

1. Lead efforts to review, evaluate, and improve veterinary medical education in order to prepare graduates with the competencies needed to address societal needs.
2. Lead efforts to increase the amount of veterinary research conducted and the number of graduates entering research careers.
3. Lead efforts to recruit a student body aligned with the demands for veterinary expertise.
4. Lead efforts to increase the number of racially and/or ethnically underrepresented in veterinary medicine (URVM*) individuals throughout academic veterinary medicine.
5. Lead efforts to develop the next generation of leaders for academic veterinary medicine.
6. Strengthen AAVMC's capacity to better serve its members, partners, and other stakeholders in advancing the AAVMC mission.

*"URVMs are populations of individuals whose advancement in the veterinary medical profession have historically been disproportionately impacted by six specific aspects of diversity (gender, race, ethnicity, and geographic, socio-economic, and educational disadvantage) due to legal, cultural, or social climate impediments." *Definition of Underrepresented in Veterinary Medicine (URVM)*, approved by the AAVMC Board of Directors, July 20, 2008.

*Left: A Tufts University Cummings School of Veterinary Medicine student checks out a horse with advice from her professor. Photo courtesy of Andy Cunningham of the Tufts University Cummings School of Veterinary Medicine.*

# VETERINARY MEDICINE: OPPORTUNITIES AND CHOICES

Veterinarians help animals and people live longer, healthier lives. They serve society through the protection of animal health and welfare, the prevention and relief of animal suffering, the conservation of animal resources, the promotion of public health, and the advancement of medical knowledge. The Doctor of Veterinary Medicine degree can lead to diverse career opportunities and different lifestyles from a solo mixed-animal practice in a rural area to a teaching or research position at an urban university, medical center, or industrial laboratory. The majority of veterinarians in the United States are in private clinical practice, although significant numbers are involved in preventive medicine, regulatory veterinary medicine, military veterinary medicine, laboratory animal medicine, research and development in industry, and teaching and research in a variety of basic science and clinical disciplines.

## THE SPECTRUM OF OPPORTUNITIES IN VETERINARY MEDICINE

Veterinarians may choose to become specialists in a clinical area or to work with particular species. The first step on the path toward specialization is usually an internship.

### 1) FURTHER TRAINING

#### Internship

Internships are one-year programs in either small- or large-animal medicine and surgery. The most prestigious internship programs are at veterinary medical colleges or at very large private veterinary hospitals with board-certified veterinarians on staff. Since internships are usually at large referral centers, interns are exposed to a larger number of challenging cases than they would be likely to see in a smaller private practice.

Veterinary students in their senior year and veterinary graduates apply for internships through a matching program. Internship applicants and training hospitals rank each other in order of preference, and a computerized system matches each applicant with the highest-ranking teaching hospital that ranked the applicant. Academic performance in the veterinary professional curriculum, as well as recommendations from veterinary school faculty, is considered in the ranking of internship applicants.

Most veterinary interns in the United States receive a nominal salary, and their educational debts, if any, may be postponed in some governmentally subsidized loan programs. Veterinarians can sometimes command a higher starting salary in private practice after completion of an internship. Also, an internship is often the next step, after receiving the veterinary degree, toward residency and board certification.

#### Residency Training

Residency training is more specialized than an internship. Residency training programs are competitive and most require that the prospective residents complete an internship or equivalent private-practice experience prior to beginning the residency programs. Residency training is available in disciplines as varied as internal medicine, surgery, preventive medicine, behavior, toxicology, dentistry, and pathology.

The programs take two to three years to complete, depending on the nature of the specialty. Successful completion of a residency often is an important step toward attainment of board certification. Some residencies combine research and graduate study, leading to master's or PhD degrees.

#### Board Certification

Currently, there are twenty-two AVMA-recognized veterinary specialty organizations, comprising forty distinct specialties: anesthesiology, animal behavior, clinical pharmacology, dentistry, dermatology, emergency and critical care, internal medicine, laboratory animal medicine, microbiology, nutrition, ophthalmology, pathology, poultry medicine, private practice, preventive medicine, radiology, surgery, sports medicine and rehabilitation, theriogenology (reproduction), toxicology, and zoological medicine. Veterinarians may become board certified by completing rigorous postgraduate training, education, and examination requirements.

### 2) PRIVATE AND PUBLIC PRACTICE

The majority of veterinary graduates are engaged in private practice, either as an owner of a solo practice or, more likely, as a partner or associate in a group practice. Increasingly, veterinarians work together as a team, which allows a wider range of services to be provided.

Small-animal veterinarians focus their efforts primarily on dogs and cats but are seeing a growing number of other pets, including other small mammals, birds, reptiles, and fish.

Large-animal veterinarians often place their emphasis on horses, cattle, or pigs, and work both on a farm-call and an in-clinic basis. A mixed-animal veterinarian works with all types of domestic animals.

Public practice provides a variety of opportunities at the international, national, state, county, or city levels. There are exciting career opportunities for veterinarians in food safety, public health, the military, animal disease control, and research. Some veterinarians are employed by zoos and aquariums, wildlife conservation groups, game farms, or fisheries.

## 3) INDUSTRY

Veterinarians have many opportunities available to them in private industry, particularly in the fields of nutrition and pharmaceuticals. Assisting in the development of new products in the animal industry, conducting research for pharmaceutical companies, diagnosing disease and drug effects as pathologists, or safeguarding the health of laboratory animal colonies are all interesting career possibilities.

## 4) CONCLUSION

By the very nature of the comparative medical education that veterinarians receive, the many species of animals they care for and work for, and the wide variety of clientele served, the opportunities available to today's veterinarian are abundant.

# INFORMATION ABOUT STANDARDIZED TESTS

Most veterinary medical colleges require one or more standardized tests: the Graduate Record Examination (GRE) or the Medical College Admission Test (MCAT). For further information regarding test dates and registration procedures, contact the testing agencies listed below:

GRE Graduate Record Examinations
P.O. Box 6000
Princeton, NJ 08541-6000
(609) 771-7670 (Princeton, NJ)
also: (510) 654-1200 (Oakland, CA)
www.gre.org
Individual school codes: see GRE booklet

MCAT Medical College Admission Test
MCAT Program Office
P.O. Box 4056
Iowa City, IA 52243-4056
(319) 337-1357
www.aamc.org/students/applying/mcat

TOEFL Test of English as a Foreign Language
TOEFL/TSE Services
P.O. Box 6151
Princeton, NJ 08541-6151
(609) 771-7100
www.toefl.org

# AAVMC MEMBER INSTITUTIONS AND THE ROLE OF ACCREDITATION

Veterinary Schools join the AAVMC as institutional or affiliate members. A key difference between these two membership categories is whether a college/school of veterinary medicine is accredited by the American Veterinary Medical Association's Council on Education (AVMA/COE). Only AVMA/COE-accredited colleges of veterinary medicine may join AAVMC as an institutional (voting) member. Colleges of veterinary medicine that are not AVMA-accredited may join AAVMC as an affiliate member (non-voting) only. Several of AAVMC's affiliate members (non-AVMA/COE-accredited institutions) have entered into agreements with AAVMC institutional members for clinical training. It is important for prospective veterinary students to know the different implications of attending and/or graduating from AVMA/COE-accredited vs. non-AVMA/COE-accredited colleges of veterinary medicine as it pertains to educational options and eventually seeking and obtaining a license to practice veterinary medicine. AAVMC encourages its affiliate members to become AVMA/COE-accredited.

## ACCREDITATION

The AVMA/COE accredits DVM or equivalent educational programs. Accreditation through the AVMA/COE assures that minimum standards in veterinary medical education are met by accredited colleges of veterinary medicine and that students enrolled in these colleges receive an education that will prepare them for entry-level positions in the profession. In the United States, graduation from an AVMA/COE-accredited college of veterinary medicine is an important prerequisite for application for licensure. Internationally, some veterinary schools have chosen to seek AVMA/COE accreditation in addition to accreditation by the competent authority in their own regions. AVMA/COE accreditation of international veterinary schools provides assurance that those programs of education meet the same standards as other similarly accredited schools.

Additionally, AVMA/COE accreditation assures:
- Prospective students that they will meet a competency threshold for entry into practice, including eligibility for professional credentialing and/or licensure;
- Employers that graduates have achieved specified learning goals and are prepared to begin professional practice;
- Faculty, deans, and administrators that their programs measure satisfactorily against national standards and their own stated missions and goals;
- The public that public health and safety concerns are being addressed; and
- The veterinary profession that the science and art of veterinary medicine are being advanced through contemporary curricula.

*Source: The source for this information and a site recommended for obtaining additional information is as follows: www.avma.org/education/cvea/about_accred.asp

## LICENSURE

### Licensure in the United States

In the United States, requirements for licensure are set by individual state regulatory boards. The North American Veterinary Licensing Exam (NAVLE) and any additional state exams must be taken by a graduate to become eligible for state licensure. The NAVLE, which is administered by the National Board of Veterinary Medical Examiners (NBVME), fulfills a core requirement for licensure to practice veterinary medicine in all jurisdictions in the United States and Canada. Mexico does not require NAVLE. In addition to the NAVLE, state regulatory boards will have other licensure requirements, which may include state-specific examinations.

To be eligible to take the NAVLE, applicants must have graduated from either an AVMA/COE-accredited college of veterinary medicine or a non-AVMA/COE-accredited college (see following details).

Applicants who graduated from a non-AVME/COE-accredited college must also have a certification of eligibility, which can come from one of two sources: the Educational Commission for Foreign Veterinary Graduates (ECFVG) Certification Program (www.avma.org/professionaldevelopment/education/foreign/pages/default.aspx) or the Program for the Assessment of Veterinary Education Equivalence (PAVE) (www.aavsb.org/PAVE).

All state regulatory boards accept the ECFVG certification, administered through the AVMA, as meeting in full or in part the educational prerequisite for licensure eligibility. At this time, twenty-eight state regulatory boards also accept PAVE certification, which is administered through the American Association of Veterinary State Boards (AAVSB).

It is important to note that prerequisites for licensure eligibility and requirements for licensure vary amongst state regulatory boards and are subject to periodic modification.

## Licensure Outside the United States

Mutual recognition arrangements apply to jurisdictions where there are AVMA/COE-accredited schools. These specify that graduates of AVMA/COE-accredited schools in the United States and Canada are permitted to obtain licensure to practice under terms no less favorable than graduates of schools accredited by the competent authority in that jurisdiction.

## DECIDING WHERE TO APPLY

There are several factors, as well as the issue of accreditation, that an applicant must consider in identifying school(s) to submit an application for admissions. In addition to licensure issues, there may be economic, educational options, or other differences that students should consider in making decisions on where to apply. This book is intended to provide important information about AAVMC members to assist in informed decision-making for students considering applying to one or more veterinary colleges.

# VETERINARIAN PROFILE: ANTHONY HALL

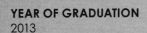

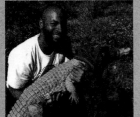

**YEAR OF GRADUATION**
2013

**PLACE OF EMPLOYMENT**
Banfield Pet Hospital

**What is your favorite aspect of being a veterinarian?**
Being able to treat pets for the myriad of conditions they present with, as well as educating the client on how to properly take care of his or her animal, while strengthening the human-animal bond at the same time.

**What type of veterinary medicine do you practice?**
General medicine and surgery.

**Where did you attend veterinary school?**
Ross University School of Veterinary Medicine (RUSVM) and Virginia-Maryland Regional College of Veterinary Medicine (VMRCVM).

**How long have you been practicing as a veterinarian?**
Since November 2013.

**What advice do you have for those considering a career in veterinary medicine?**
Test it out first to make sure it's something you really want to do. It is not glamorous, and can be hazardous and hard work. You have to have a passion and drive for this. Volunteer at a shelter or clinic to see if you can handle not just the cute puppies and kittens, but some of the serious, more challenging and unappealing cases.

**What challenges have you faced while practicing veterinary medicine?**
As a new grad, facing clients and gaining the confidence of putting my years of schooling to actual use.

**What is your proudest moment of your veterinary career so far?**
So far, it would be seeing the face of a client after you've told them that the cancerous growth you removed had clean margins.

**What led you to pursue a career in veterinary medicine?**
I suppose an inner drive. Ever since I was four, I said I'd be a vet. And now I am. I never had a doubt that this is what I want to do, and I considered (but didn't follow through with) only one other option for career.

# GEOGRAPHICAL LISTING OF AAVMC INSTITUTIONAL (AVMA/COE ACCREDITED) VETERINARY SCHOOLS AND DIRECTORY OF ADMISSIONS OFFICES

## UNITED STATES

### ALABAMA

Auburn University
Office for Academic Affairs
College of Veterinary Medicine
217 Goodwin/Overton
Auburn, AL 36849-5536

Tuskegee University
Office of Admissions and
    Recruitment
School of Veterinary Medicine
100 Dr. Frederick Patterson Hall
Tuskegee, AL 36088

### ARIZONA

Midwestern University
College of Veterinary Medicine
19555 North 59th Avenue
Glendale, AZ 85308

### CALIFORNIA

University of California
School of Veterinary Medicine
Office of the Dean-Student
    Programs
One Shields Avenue
Davis, CA 95616

Western University of Health
    Sciences
Office of Admissions
College of Veterinary Medicine
309 East 2nd Street
Pomona, CA 91766-1854

### COLORADO

Colorado State University
College of Veterinary Medicine and
    Biomedical Sciences
1601 Campus Delivery – Office of
    the Dean
Fort Collins, CO 80523-1601

### FLORIDA

University of Florida
Admissions Office
College of Veterinary Medicine
P.O. Box 100125
Gainesville, FL 32610-0125

### GEORGIA

The University of Georgia
Admissions Department
Office for Academic Affairs
College of Veterinary Medicine
Athens, GA 30602-7372

### ILLINOIS

University of Illinois
College of Veterinary Medicine
Office of Academic and Student
    Affairs
2001 South Lincoln Avenue,
    Room 2271g
Urbana, IL 61802

### INDIANA

Purdue University
Student Services Center
College of Veterinary Medicine
625 Harrison Street
West Lafayette, IN 47907-2026

### IOWA

Iowa State University
Office of Admissions
College of Veterinary Medicine
2270 Veterinary Medicine
P.O. Box 3020
Ames, IA 50010-3020

### KANSAS

Kansas State University
Office of Admissions
College of Veterinary Medicine
101 Trotter Hall
Manhattan, KS 66506-5601

### LOUISIANA

Louisiana State University
Office of Student and Academic Affairs
School of Veterinary Medicine
Skip Bertman Drive
Baton Rouge, LA 70803

### MASSACHUSETTS

Tufts University
Office of Admissions
Cummings School of Veterinary
    Medicine
200 Westboro Road
North Grafton, MA 01536

### MICHIGAN

Michigan State University
Office of Admissions
College of Veterinary Medicine
784 Wilson Road
F-110 Veterinary Medical Center
East Lansing, MI 48824

### MINNESOTA

University of Minnesota
Office of Academic and Student Affairs
College of Veterinary Medicine
108 Pomeroy Center
1964 Fitch Ave.
St. Paul, MN 55108

### MISSISSIPPI

Mississippi State University
Office of Student Admissions
College of Veterinary Medicine
P.O. Box 6100
Mississippi State, MS 39762

### MISSOURI

University of Missouri-Columbia
Office of Academic Affairs
College of Veterinary Medicine
W203 Veterinary Medicine Building
Columbia, MO 65211

## NEW YORK

Cornell University
Office of Student & Academic Services
College of Veterinary Medicine
S2-009 Schurman Hall
Ithaca, NY 14853-6401

## NORTH CAROLINA

North Carolina State University
Student Services Office
College of Veterinary Medicine
1060 William Moore Drive, Box 8401
Raleigh, NC 27607

## OHIO

The Ohio State University
Office of Student Affairs
College of Veterinary Medicine
Suite 127 Veterinary Medicine
   Academic Building
1900 Coffey Road
Columbus, OH 43210-1089

## OKLAHOMA

Oklahoma State University
Office of Admissions
112 McElroy Hall
Center for Veterinary Health
   Sciences
College of Veterinary Medicine
Stillwater, OK 74078-2003

## OREGON

Oregon State University
Office of the Dean
Attention: Admissions
College of Veterinary Medicine
200 Magruder Hall
Corvallis, OR 97331-4801

## PENNSYLVANIA

University of Pennsylvania
Admissions Office
School of Veterinary Medicine
3800 Spruce Street
Philadelphia, PA 19104-6044

## TENNESSEE

Lincoln Memorial University
College of Veterinary Medicine
6965 Cumberland Gap Pkway
Harrogate, TN 37752

The University of Tennessee
Admissions Office
College of Veterinary Medicine
2407 River Drive
Room A-104-C
Knoxville, TN 37996-4550

## TEXAS

Texas A & M University
Office of the Dean
College of Veterinary Medicine
   & Biomedical Sciences
College Station, TX 77843-4461

## VIRGINIA

Virginia-Maryland Regional College
   of Veterinary Medicine
Admissions Coordinator
Blacksburg, VA 24061

## WASHINGTON

Washington State University
Office of Student Services
College of Veterinary Medicine
100 Grimes Way
P.O. Box 647012
Pullman, WA 99164-7012

## WISCONSIN

University of Wisconsin-Madison
Office of Academic Affairs
School of Veterinary Medicine
2015 Linden Drive
Madison, WI 53706-1102

# INTERNATIONAL

## AUSTRALIA

Murdoch University
Murdoch International
South Street
Murdoch 6150
Western Australia

University of Melbourne
Faculty of Veterinary Science
Corner Park Drive and
   Flemington Road
Parkville
Melbourne 3010
Victoria Australia

University of Queensland–Gatton
   Campus
School of Veterinary Science
Gatton, 4343
Queensland, Australia
University of Sydney
Faculty of Veterinary Science
Sydney, NSW 2006
Australia

School of Veterinary Science
University of Queensland–Gatton
   Campus
Gatton, 4343
Queensland, Australia

## CANADA

### ALBERTA

University of Calgary
Admissions Office
Faculty of Veterinary Medicine
TRW 2D03
3280 Hospital Drive NW
Calgary, AB T2N 4Z6

### MONTRÉAL

Université de Montréal
Service des Admissions
C.P. 6205
Succursale Centre-Ville
Montréal Québec H3C 3T5 Canada

### ONTARIO

University of Guelph
Admissions Services
University Centre, Level 3
Guelph Ontario N 1G 2W 1
Canada

### PRINCE EDWARD ISLAND

University of Prince Edward Island
Registrar's Office
Atlantic Veterinary College
550 University Avenue
Charlottetown PEI C1A 4P3
Canada

## SASKATCHEWAN

University of Saskatchewan
Admissions Office
Western College of Veterinary
  Medicine
52 Campus Drive
Saskatoon Saskatchewan S7N 5B4
Canada

## CARIBBEAN

Ross University School of Veterinary
  Medicine
Office of Admissions
630 US HWY 1
North Brunswick, NJ 08902

St. George's University
Office of Admission
St. George's University
c/o The North American
  Correspondent
University Support Services, LLC
3500 Sunrise Highway
Building 300
Great River, NY 11739

## ENGLAND

Royal Veterinary College
Head of Admissions
Royal College Street
London NW1 0TU
England

## IRELAND

University College Dublin
Veterinary Medicine Applications
UCD Admissions Office
Tierney Building
Belfield, Dublin 4
Ireland

## MEXICO

Universidad Nacional Autónoma de
  México
Office of Undergraduate
  Studies (Division de Estudios
  Profesionales)
College of Veterinary Medicine
  (FMVZ)
Av. Universidad 3000
Circuito Interior
Delegacion Coyoacan
Mexico D.F. 04510

## THE NETHERLANDS

Utrecht University
Office for International Cooperation
Faculty of Veterinary Medicine
Yalelaan 1
3584 CL Utrecht
The Netherlands

## NEW ZEALAND

Massey University Veterinary School
International Student Affairs
Undergraduate Office
IVABS
Massey University
Private Bag 11-222
Palmerston North 4442
New Zealand

## SCOTLAND

The University of Edinburgh
Admissions Office
Royal (Dick) School of Veterinary
  Studies
Easter Bush Veterinary Centre
Roslin EH25 9RG
Scotland

University of Glasgow
Director of Admissions & Student
  Services Manager
College of Medicine, Veterinary and
  Life Sciences
School of Veterinary Medicine
  Undergraduate School
464 Bearsden Road
Glasgow G61 1QH

# GEOGRAPHICAL LISTING OF AAVMC AFFILIATE (NON-AVMA/COE ACCREDITED) VETERINARY SCHOOLS AND DIRECTORY OF ADMISSIONS OFFICES

## CARIBBEAN

St. Matthew's University
Office of Admissions
12124 High Tech Avenue,
Suite 350
Orlando, Fl 32817

## COSTA RICA

1 Km al Oeste de Casa Presidencial
San José 10105
Costa Rica

## DENMARK

University of Copenhagen
Office for International Cooperation
Faculty of Health and Medicine
Blegdamsvej 3B
DK-2200 Copenhagen N
Denmark

## JAPAN

University of Tokyo
Tokyo 113-8657
Japan

## PHILIPPINES

Central Luzon State University
   Science City of Munoz
Nueva Ecija 3120
Philippines

# LISTING OF CONTRACTING STATES AND PROVINCES

Six Canadian provinces and 19 states in the United States have a veterinary school contract with one or more schools to provide access to veterinary medical education for their residents. The state or province, working through the contracting agency, usually agrees to pay a fee to help cover the cost of education for a certain number of places in each entering class. Residents from the contract states then compete with each other for those positions.

Some states contract with more than one school. For example, Arkansas contracts with 5 veterinary schools, and North Dakota contracts with 6 schools. Connecticut, Rhode Island, Vermont, Nebraska, and the District of Columbia presently have no contracts, so all candidates from these places apply as nonresidents to veterinary schools of their choice.

The educational agreements between contracting agencies and veterinary schools differ. Under some contract arrangements, students pay in-state tuition; in others, they pay nonresident tuition. Some contract states require students to repay all or part of the subsidy that the state provided; others require veterinary graduates to return to practice in the state for a period of time. Applicants should be aware of their obligation to the state before agreeing to participate in a contract program.

Following is a list of states and provinces that have educational agreements with schools of veterinary medicine.

## UNITED STATES

### ARIZONA

Contracts through WICHE* with University of California, Colorado State University, Oregon State University, and Washington State University.

### ARKANSAS

Contracts in past with Louisiana State University, University of Missouri, and Oklahoma State University. Contracts not all completed at time of printing; may be some changes.

### CONNECTICUT

Contracts with Iowa State University.

### DELAWARE

Contracts with Oklahoma State University and the University of Georgia.

### HAWAII

Contracts through WICHE* with University of California, Colorado State University, Oregon State University, and Washington State University.

### IDAHO

Contracts with Washington State University.

### KENTUCKY

Contracts with Auburn University and Tuskegee University.

### MONTANA

Contracts through WICHE* with University of California, Colorado State University, Oregon State University, and Washington State University.

### NEBRASKA

Formal education alliance with Iowa State University.

### NEVADA

Contracts through WICHE* with University of California, Colorado State University, Oregon State University, and Washington State University.

### NEW MEXICO

Contracts through WICHE* with University of California, Colorado State University, Oregon State University, and Washington State University.

### NORTH DAKOTA

Contracts with Iowa State University, Kansas State University, and the University of Minnesota. Contracts through WICHE* with the University of California, Colorado State University, Oregon State University, and Washington State University.

### SOUTH CAROLINA

Contracts with University of Georgia , Mississippi State University, and Tuskegee University.

### SOUTH DAKOTA

Reciprocity with University of Minnesota. Contracts with Iowa State University.

### UTAH

Contracts through WICHE* with University of California, Colorado State University, and Oregon State University. Contracts with Washington State University.

* WICHE = Western Interstate Commission for Higher Education (offices in Boulder, Colorado)

## WEST VIRGINIA

Contracts with Tuskegee University, Mississippi State University, Auburn University, and Virginia-Maryland Regional College of Veterinary Medicine.

## WYOMING

Contracts through WICHE* with the University of California, Colorado State University, Oregon State University, and Washington State University.

# CANADA

## ALBERTA

Contracts with University of Saskatchewan and University of Calgary.

## BRITISH COLUMBIA

Contracts with University of Saskatchewan.

## MANITOBA

Contracts with University of Saskatchewan.

## NEW BRUNSWICK

Contracts with Atlantic Veterinary College at the University of Prince Edward Island and Université de Montréal.

## NEWFOUNDLAND

Contracts with Atlantic Veterinary College at the University of Prince Edward Island.

## NOVA SCOTIA

Contracts with Atlantic Veterinary College at the University of Prince Edward Island.

---

* WICHE = Western Interstate Commission for Higher Education (offices in Boulder, Colorado)

# PROGRAMS FOR MULTICULTURAL OR DISADVANTAGED STUDENTS

The Association of American Veterinary Medical Colleges affirms the value of diversity within the veterinary medical profession. The membership is committed to incorporating that belief into their actions by advocating for the recruitment and retention of underrepresented persons as students and faculty, and ultimately fostering their success in the profession of veterinary medicine. The Association believes that through these actions, society and the profession will be well served.

Many schools have programs designed to facilitate entry into, and retention by, veterinary programs nationwide. These programs are directed at several levels, from high-school students to the student who has already been accepted by a veterinary college. Most of these programs will accept students from every state, regardless of the school(s) to which an individual might eventually apply or attend.

Following is an alphabetical list of schools by state and a short explanation of their programs:

## UNIVERSITY OF CALIFORNIA

*Program:* Summer Enrichment Program
*Description:* a 6-week summer program. The purpose of this program is to increase the academic preparedness of disadvantaged students through science-based learning skills development, clinical education, individual advising, and student development.
*Eligibility:* Educationally and/or economically disadvantaged. Must have completed at least one year of college with a minimum science GPA of 2.8 and demonstrated interest in veterinary medicine.
*Program dates:* July–August.
*Contact:* Office of the Dean–Student Programs, School of Veterinary Medicine, University of California, One Shields Avenue, Davis CA 95616; telephone: (530) 752-1383.
*Sponsorship:* School of Veterinary Medicine, University of California-Davis.

## COLORADO STATE UNIVERSITY

*Program:* Vet Prep
*Description:* a one-year academic program that serves as a bridge to the professional veterinary medical program for disadvantaged (cultural, social, economic) applicants who ranked high but were denied admission during the current admissions process. Limited to 10 students who upon successful completion are guaranteed admission to the veterinary program. Candidates are selected from the current regular admissions applicant pool.
*Eligibility:* disadvantaged students.
*Contact:* College of Veterinary Medicine and Biomedical Sciences, W102 Anatomy, Colorado State University, Fort Collins CO 80523; telephone: (970) 491-7051; email: DVMAdmissions@colostate.edu.
*Sponsorship:* College of Veterinary Medicine and Biomedical Sciences, Colorado State University.

*Program:* Vet Start
*Description:* an 8-year undergraduate and professional program for students who enter Colorado State from high school resulting in a bachelor's and a professional degree. Undergraduate and professional program scholarships are provided, and admission to the professional veterinary medical program is guaranteed upon successful completion of the undergraduate requirements. Mentoring, support services, and summer jobs are available to participants.
*Eligibility:* students who have a disadvantaged background (economic, cultural, or social) will be given special consideration. Students must be high-school graduates with fewer than 15 semester credits of college coursework post high school graduation. Selection is competitive. There are 5 positions per year for incoming freshman undergraduate students.
*Program dates:* begins fall semester; applications available online early December; application deadline typically March 1.
*Contact:* College of Veterinary Medicine and Biomedical Sciences, Campus Delivery 1601, Colorado State University, Fort Collins CO 80523-1601; telephone: (970) 491-7051; email: ken.blehm@colostate.edu.
*Sponsorship:* College of Veterinary Medicine and Biomedical Sciences, Colorado State University.

## CORNELL UNIVERSITY

*Program:* State University of New York Graduate Underrepresented Minority Fellowships
*Description:* all matriculating underrepresented minorities are eligible (not restricted by state residency).
*Contact:* Director of Student Financial Planning, Office of Student & Academic Services, College of Veterinary Medicine, Cornell University, S2-009 Schurman Hall, Ithaca NY 14853-6401; telephone: (607) 253-3766; www.vet.cornell.edu/financialaid/.

## MICHIGAN STATE UNIVERSITY

*Program:* Vetward Bound Program

*Description:* Vetward Bound offers different levels of programming, each with its own eligibility requirements. The program provides a review of basic science content, research and/or clinical experience, preparation for the GRE, veterinary experience, food and fiber animal experience, study strategy development, and field experiences. Level placement is determined by program staff and is based on educational background.

*Eligibility:* Economically and educationally disadvantaged first year undergraduate students through prematriculants into the professional degree program. Students selected to participate will meet HHS Health Careers Opportunity Program guidelines and Federal thresholds. An individual will be determined to be disadvantaged if he or she comes from a background that has inhibited the individual from obtaining the knowledge, skills, and abilities required to enroll in and graduate from a health professions school or comes from a family with an annual income below a level based on low income thresholds according to family size published by the Bureau of the Census, adjusted annually for changes in the Consumer Price Index, and adjusted by the Secretary for use in health professions programs.

*Program dates:* June–July.

*Contact:* Vetward Bound Coordinator, College of Veterinary Medicine, 784 Wilson Road, F-110 Veterinary Medical Center, Michigan State University, East Lansing MI 48824; telephone: (517) 355-6521; email: vetbound@cvm.msu.edu.

## MISSISSIPPI STATE UNIVERSITY

*Program:* Board of Trustees of State Institutions of Higher Learning Veterinary Medicine Minority Loan/Scholarship Program

*Description:* a financial assistance program for Mississippi residents who are underrepresented minorities. The loan to service obligation is one year for each year of scholarship assistance, not to exceed four years.

*Contact:* Susan Eckels, Program Administrator, Mississippi Institutions of Higher Learning, 3825 Ridgewood Road, Jackson MS 39211-6453; telephone: (800) 327-2980.

## NORTH CAROLINA STATE UNIVERSITY

*Program:* UNC Campus Scholarship Program—Graduate Student Component

*Description:* UNC General Administration funds this program. Eligibility is limited to new or continuing full-time doctoral students who have financial need and who are residents of North Carolina as of the beginning of the award period (as determined under the *Manual to Assist the Public Higher Education Institutions of N.C. in the Matter of Student Resident Classification for Tuition Purposes*). Individuals who have been accepted to a master's degree program in a department offering the doctoral degree and who intend, and will be eligible, to pursue doctoral studies at NC State after completion of the requirements for the master's degree are also eligible. The program provides up to $3,000 annually for North Carolina residents.

*Contact:* Director of Diversity Affairs, College of Veterinary Medicine, North Carolina State University, 1060 William Moore Drive, Box 8401, Raleigh, NC 27607; telephone: (919) 513-6262; website: www.cvm.ncsu.edu.

*Program:* Diversity Graduate Assistant Grant

*Description:* Funded by the North Carolina State University Graduate School, recipients must be full-time, new or continuing students pursuing master's and doctoral degrees at North Carolina State University. The program provides up to $3,000 annually. Both resident and nonresident students are eligible to apply.

*Contact:* Director of Diversity Affairs, College of Veterinary Medicine, North Carolina State University, 1060 William Moore Drive, Box 8401, Raleigh, NC 27607; telephone: (919) 513-6262; website: www.cvm.ncsu.edu.

*Note:* North Carolina residents are encouraged to apply for both programs. However, the annual maximum award for these grant programs is a combined $3,000 (with an option of $500 in additional support for study in the summer). The grant is awarded on an annual basis. Awardees must reapply each year.

## THE OHIO STATE UNIVERSITY

*Program:* Young Scholars Program

*Description:* this summer program is offered to seventh- through eleventh-grade students from Ohio. It provides hands-on science activities, academic enrichment exercises, and career exploration opportunities.

*Eligibility:* disadvantaged students recommended by their faculty.

*Program dates:* June to August each summer.

*Sponsorship:* the State of Ohio and The Ohio State University.

*Program:* Summer Research Opportunity Program

*Description:* this program is designed to promote the migration of minority undergraduate students into graduate research educational programs by providing them with summer research experiences. The student is provided with his or her individualized research problem by a faculty mentor and expected to carry that research through to publication.

*Eligibility:* the student must have completed 2 years of college work and have achieved at least a 2.50 cumulative GPA. The student must be an underrepresented minority or economically disadvantaged.

*Contact:* Graduate School, The Ohio State University, 230 North Oval Mall, Columbus OH 43210.

*Sponsorship:* the Big Ten Consortium for Institutional Studies.

## PURDUE UNIVERSITY

*Program:* Access to Animal-Related Careers (A²RC)

*Description:* A²RC is a two-week, residential program offering hands-on experiences in multiple areas of veterinary medicine including swine production medicine, small animal medicine, and equine medicine. Also included are sessions on several specialty areas such as cardiology, emergency and critical care medicine, and radiology. The program is designed to expose participants to life as a first year DVM student. Mock admissions interviews are conducted and participants are given individual feedback.

*Eligibility:* A²RC is targeted to 2nd and 3rd year underrepresented minority undergraduate students at partner institutions enrolled in pre-veterinary studies.

*Program dates:* May 18–June 1, 2014

For more information on the A²RC program, and to obtain an application, please contact the PVM Director of Diversity Initiatives (contact information below).

*Contact:* Dr. Kauline Cipriani Davis, Director of Diversity Initiatives (ciprianik@purdue.edu or 765 496-1940; website http://www.vet.purdue.edu/diversity/index.php)

## UNIVERSITY OF TENNESSEE

*Program:* Veterinary Summer Experience for Tennessee High School Students

*Description:* The College of Veterinary Medicine offers an eight-week program that provides high school students an opportunity to gain experience working with veterinarians at a veterinary practice in their home towns for seven weeks during the summer. During the eighth week of this summer experience, students will be guests of the College of Veterinary Medicine on the campus of The University of Tennessee in Knoxville. Students will attend clinical rotations in the Equine, Farm Animal, Small Animal, and Avian and Exotic Animal (including zoo medicine) Hospitals in the Veterinary Medical Center.

Students will also attend special educational functions related to veterinary medicine.

*Eligibility:* To qualify for this summer program, a student must be a Tennessee resident and be at least 16 years of age by June 1, be enrolled as a senior or junior in a Tennessee high school, and have earned a minimum 3.0 high school GPA. Applicants must also have an interest in veterinary medicine as a potential career. Preference will be given to applicants who will contribute greatly to the diversity of the summer program and, potentially, to the veterinary profession. Students receive a financial stipend for satisfactory performance in the eight-week program.

*Program dates:* Summer

*Contact:* Dr. William Hill, The University of Tennessee, College of Veterinary Medicine, 2431 Joe Johnson Drive, 339 Ellington Plant Science, Knoxville TN 37996, telephone: (865) 974-5770. E-mail: wahill@utk.edu.

## UNIVERSITY OF MINNESOTA

*Program:* Veterinary Leadership in Early Admissions for Diversity (VetLEAD)

*Description:* VetLEAD creates a pathway into the DVM program for high-ability students at under-represented serving partner schools, including Florida Agricultural and Mechanical University (FAMU).

*Eligibility:* Any high-achieving student enrolled in the Animal Science program at FAMU may apply for an early admissions decision at the end of their sophomore year of undergraduate studies. Eligible students have past experience working or volunteering in a veterinary related setting, a FAMU cumulative GPA of 3.4 with coursework consistent with required prerequisite courses, and strong letters of references.

*Contact:* Karen Nelson, Director of Admissions, dvminfo@umn.edu

## TUSKEGEE UNIVERSITY

*Program:* Summer Enrichment and Reinforcement Program (SERP) Description: this 6-week preadmission program is designed to provide academic enrichment through effective learning strategies and mentorship to facilitate the entry of "at risk" students into the veterinary program and successful transition through the professional curriculum.

*Description:* this 8-week preadmission activity is designed to facilitate the entry of "at risk" students and provide the skills necessary for successful transition to the professional school.

*Eligibility:* participation is targeted to minority and disadvantaged students who have completed at least 3

years of college and all preveterinary prerequisites. Participation is restricted to persons who have applied to the DVM program in the College of Veterinary Medicine, Nursing, and Allied Health and who have been recommended by the Veterinary Admissions Committee for evaluation to the program.

*Program dates:* the summer before fall semester.

*Contact:* Associate Dean for Academic Affairs, College of Veterinary Medicine, Nursing and Allied Health, Tuskegee University, Tuskegee, AL 36088.

*Sponsorship:* this program is sponsored by a grant from the U.S. Department of Health and Human Services.

*Program:* Veterinary Science Training, Education and Preparation Institutes for Minority Students (Vet-Step I and II)

*Description:* Consists of 2 one-week programs designed to encourage high achieving minority students to consider veterinary medicine as a career choice. The program focus on progressive learning skills in reading comprehension, study skills, time-management, note-taking, medical vocabulary, etc.

*Eligibility:* Vet-Step I accepts 30 students from grades 9 and 10; Vet-Step II accepts students from Vet-Step I and from grade 12. Minority high school honor students interested in the biomedical sciences are strongly encouraged to apply.

*Contact:* Coordinator, Vet-Step Program, College of Veterinary Medicine, Nursing, and Allied Health, Tuskegee University, Tuskegee AL 36088, (334) 727-8309.

*Sponsorship:* U.S. Department of Health and Human Services.

## VIRGINIA-MARYLAND REGIONAL COLLEGE OF VETERINARY MEDICINE

*Program:* Multicultural Academic Opportunities Program

*Description:* a 10-week program providing opportunities to conduct scientific research; participate in clinical rotations within the veterinary teaching hospital; improve leadership, public speaking, and self-marketing skills; attend GRE preparatory classes; and learn about admission into graduate / professional school.

*Contact:* Admissions Office at Blacksburg campus.

*Program:* Summer Research Apprenticeship Program—College Park

*Description:* a summer research program providing research experience to veterinary and preveterinary students from diverse backgrounds, including economic hardship and underrepresented racial/ethnic groups. Projects may include assisting in the planning, preparation, and data collection for controlled experiments, clinical trials, or epidemiological investigations; researching disease processes; and performing literature searches.

*Contact:* Admissions Office at College Park campus.

*Scholarship Opportunities:* a limited number of scholarships are available to assist minority DVM students.

## WASHINGTON STATE UNIVERSITY

*Program:* Short-Term Research Training Program for Veterinary Students

*Description:* a 3-month summer program designed to promote interest in research by veterinary students. Emphasis is on a hands-on research project supervised by a faculty member with a research program. Stipends are provided.

*Eligibility:* WSU veterinary students or ethnic minority veterinary students from other U.S. colleges of veterinary medicine.

*Program dates:* 3 months in the summer dependent upon the summer vacation of the WSU College of Veterinary Medicine in which the veterinary student is enrolled.

*Contact:* Department of Veterinary Microbiology and Pathology, Washington State University, Pullman WA 99164-7040.

*Sponsorship:* The National Center for Research Resources.

## UNIVERSITY OF WISCONSIN

*Program:* Pre-College Enrollment Opportunity Program for Learning Excellence (PEOPLE)

*Description:* this program began in the summer of 1999 as a partnership between the Milwaukee Public Schools and the UW-Madison with a group of students who had just completed the ninth grade. New classes will be added each year, expanding to Madison area schools. The program is designed with a precollege track and a bridge program to undergraduate work and continues through a student's undergraduate career at University of Wisconsin-Madison. The main purposes are to promote academic preparation, increase enrollment in postsecondary institutions, and improve retention and graduation rates of minority and disadvantaged students.

*Eligibility:* students of one or more of the following ethnic heritages: African American, American Indian, Asian American, Hispanic/Latino. Other eligibility factors include economic disadvantage and current enrollment in or commitment to a college preparatory curriculum track.

*Program dates:* June–July summer residential programs and year-round nonresidential programs.

*Contact:* PEOPLE Program, 1305 Linden Drive, University of Wisconsin- Madison, Madison, WI 53706.

# FINANCIAL AID INFORMATION

Financing your veterinary medical education requires careful planning, good money management skills, and a willingness to make short-term sacrifices to achieve long-range goals.

Many of you will apply for and receive some type of financial assistance during your undergraduate education. This will help you become somewhat familiar with the process, and to know that the rules and regulations governing programs can and do change periodically.

> Don't live the lifestyle of a DVM until you have completed your education. Get in the habit of being thrifty.

As a professional student, you will be entering a partnership with the financial aid office, which will require you to complete the appropriate financial aid forms accurately, meet required deadlines, and submit any additional information that may be requested. In return, the financial aid office will determine your aid eligibility and make awards based on the available programs. Your financial aid eligibility takes into account the cost of your education minus any other available resources. Amounts of assistance and the school policies for awarding assistance vary from one veterinary medical school to another and from year to year.

Any questions or concerns that you may have about this topic need to be directed to each of the appropriate financial aid offices to ensure that you receive accurate information and guidance.

## FINANCING YOUR VETERINARY MEDICAL EDUCATION

Your education is one of the biggest investments you will make in your lifetime, and one of your most important goals should be to maximize the return on all of your investments. To reach this goal, you must take an active role in managing your financial resources. You need to understand and implement good financial practices. To get you started, here are some good financial habits you should adopt:

- Do not use credit cards to extend your lifestyle. Deciding not to use credit cards except in emergencies is one of the most important decisions you can make, and one that will reduce your stress while you are pursuing your education.

- Budget your money just as carefully as you budget your time. Contact a financial aid administrator to help you set up a budget that will be easy to follow.

- Distinguish between wants and needs. Before you make any purchase, you should ask yourself, "Do I need this, or do I want it?"

- Be a well-informed borrower. If you have not previously taken an active role in understanding the differences between various student loan programs, now is the time to do it. You need to know these differences in order to avoid high-interest loans and to borrow wisely.

- Borrow the minimum amount necessary in order to maximize the return on your educational investment.

- Be thrifty. Live as cheaply as you can. Remember, you are a student. You'll enjoy a more comfortable lifestyle once you are a DVM.

- Pay any interest that accrues on student loans if you can afford to do so, rather than let the interest accrue and capitalize. Any amount you pay while you're a student will save you money once you enter repayment.

What is the most important piece of advice for making the most of your educational investment? Don't live the lifestyle of a DVM until you have completed your education. Get in the habit of being thrifty. If you live like a DVM while you are in school, you may have to live like a student when you are a DVM.

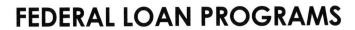

# FEDERAL LOAN PROGRAMS

Please note that subsidized loans are not available beginning fall 2012.

| | William D. Ford Unsubsidized Stafford Loan | Perkins Loan | Health Professions Student Loan | Loan for Disadvantaged Students | Grad Plus Loans for Graduate/ Professional Students |
|---|---|---|---|---|---|
| Lender | Federal Loan Program | Federal Loan Program | Federal Loan Program | Federal Loan Program | Federal Loan Program |
| Financial Need | No | Yes | Yes | Yes | No |
| Citizenship Requirement | U.S. Citizen, U.S. National, or U.S. Permanent Resident | U.S. Citizen, U.S. National, or U.S. Permanent Resident | U.S. Citizen, U.S. National, or U.S. Permanent Resident | U.S. Citizen, U.S. National, or U.S. Permanent Resident | U.S. Citizen, U.S. National, or U.S. Permanent Resident |
| Borrowing Limits | Cost of attendance minus other aid; $189,125 aggregate undergraduate and graduate | $6,000/year; $40,000 aggregate undergraduate and graduate | Cost of attendance at participating school | Federal Loan Programs | Cost of attendance minus other aid |
| Interest Rate | Fixed; capped at 6.8% | 5% | 5% | 5% | 7% |
| Interest Accrues While Enrolled in School | Yes | No | No | No | Yes |
| Deferments | Yes | Yes | Yes | Yes | Yes |
| Grace Period | Yes | Yes | Yes | Yes | No |

# A GUIDE TO PREPARING FOR VETERINARY SCHOOL

Maybe you already know that you have a strong interest in veterinary medicine, but you don't know where to start. It's never too early to begin preparing. Below are a few guidelines to help you plan your coursework and get in touch with mentors and other professionals who can help you along the way.

## HIGH SCHOOL STUDENTS

- Take science and math classes, including chemistry, biology, and algebra. If available, take Advanced Placement (AP) coursework. Note, AP courses may not always satisfy vet college prerequisite coursework, but they will give you the highest level of preparation. Consult with the vet colleges to understand if AP credit in high school will satisfy a prerequisite course requirement.
- Talk to people in the field. Call local veterinarians or contact a veterinary society in your city or town to find people who can help answer your questions.
- Gain animal experiences. These will give you a good understanding of working with animals and excellent references when you seek a volunteer experience or internship with a veterinarian. Examples include volunteering at a humane society, cleaning stables and grooming horses, doing an internship at a zoo, volunteering at a nature or wildlife center, or getting involved with 4-H, just to name a few.
- Visit veterinary college websites and perhaps make a visit during one of their admissions presentations or during an open house. The more you know early on, the better prepared you will be.
- Get on the veterinary college's mailing lists for admissions updates and invitations to programs.

## COLLEGE YEAR 1

### Fall semester

- Meet with an advisor and plan coursework. Take the list of prerequisite courses on the AAVMC website or in *VMSAR* for planning purposes. Not all vet colleges require the exact same courses, but most will want courses in the areas of biology, chemistry, and physics. That's a good place to start until you narrow down your list of vet colleges to apply to.
- Obtain a copy of the *AAVMC Veterinary Medical School Admission Requirements* (*VMSAR*) to review the veterinary schools' requirements with your advisor.
- Start working on the prerequisite coursework. Most vet colleges require quite a few biology and chemistry courses. Starting out right away in these introductory courses will allow you to move forward quickly.

### Spring semester

- Think about summer volunteer or employment opportunities in veterinary medicine, such as shadowing a veterinarian or volunteering in an animal shelter.
- Continue working on the introductory courses and register for the fall semester.
- Research preveterinary enrichment programs at ExploreHealthCareers.org. Preveterinary enrichment programs can help you decide if a career in veterinary medicine is a good fit and help prepare you for the application process.

### Summer

- Complete an internship or volunteer program.
- Attend summer school, if necessary. Note, many vet colleges prefer the prerequisite coursework be taken in a full-time load during the academic year. If possible, take general education or major courses during the summer.

## COLLEGE YEAR 2

### Fall semester

- Schedule a time to meet with your advisor.
- Attend preveterinary activities.
- Join your school's preveterinary society, if one is available.
- Continue working on prerequisite coursework.
- Explore community service opportunities through your school (they don't necessarily need to be animal-related). If possible, continue activities throughout undergraduate career.

### Spring semester

- Look into paid or volunteer veterinary-related research opportunities.
- Complete second semester coursework and register for the fall.

### Summer

- Complete a summer research or volunteer veterinary-related program.
- Attend summer school, if necessary.
- Prepare for the Graduate Record Examination (GRE).
- Visit veterinary colleges. Meet with someone from the admissions office or attend an admissions presentation and take a tour.

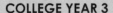

## COLLEGE YEAR 3

Fall semester

- Meet with your preveterinary advisor.
- Discuss veterinary schools.
- Register for spring semester.
- Visit the AAVMC's website (www.aavmc.org) to learn about applying to veterinary schools.
- Place your order for the *AAVMC Veterinary Medical School Admission Requirements*.
- Research schools.

Spring semester

- Identify individuals (veterinarian, faculty member or advisor, supervisor of animal experiences, research faculty) to write letters of recommendation.
- Take the GRE during late spring or early summer.
- Prepare to submit your vet school applications.
- Register for the fall semester.
- Schedule a volunteer or paid veterinary medicine-related activity.

Summer

- Take the GRE if you have not done so already.
- Budget time and finances appropriately to attend interviews.

- Participate in a volunteer or paid opportunity.
- Attend summer school, if necessary.
- Work on and submit your applications. Most vet colleges have a supplemental application, so be very careful to meet **all deadlines** for the VMCAS application, supplemental application, and getting in supporting documentation and letters.

## COLLEGE YEAR 4

Fall semester

- Meet with your advisor.
- Attend interviews with schools.
- Notification of acceptances begins December 1.

Spring semester

- Apply for federal financial aid.
- April 15 deadline to let the vet colleges where you have been admitted know your decision.

Summer

- Attend school's orientation.
- Prepare to relocate, if necessary.

# VETERINARY MEDICAL COLLEGE APPLICATION SERVICE (VMCAS)

The Veterinary Medical College Application Service is a centralized application service sponsored by the Association of American Veterinary Medical Colleges. Applicants use VMCAS to apply to most of the AVMA-accredited colleges in the United States and abroad.

VMCAS collects, processes, and ships application materials to veterinary colleges designated by the applicant, and responds to applicant inquiries about the application process. This service is the data collection, processing, and distribution component of the admission process for colleges participating in VMCAS. VMCAS, however, does not take part in the admissions selection process.

Twenty-five (25) of the twenty-eight (28) U.S. veterinary institutions participate in VMCAS, along with two (2) Canadian, two (2) Scottish, one (1) English, one (1) Irish, one (1) Australian, and one (1) New Zealand veterinary institutions. Application material deadlines, prerequisite courses, and other aspects of the admissions process differ from school to school. Applicants are responsible for being informed of all instructions provided by VMCAS and the associated member colleges. Questions about using VMCAS should be directed to the VMCAS Student and Advisor Hotline.

## APPLICATION CYCLE TIMELINE

VMCAS goes live: 1st week in June
VMCAS Application Deadline: October 2, 2014
   1:00 PM ET
Get S.E.T. for Verification: September 2, 2014*
AAVMC Acceptance Deadline: April 15, 2015
**Please be sure to verify individual school deadlines**

## KEY ONLINE RESOURCES

### General Information Chart

A one-stop comparison of school info such as location, tuition, seat availability, etc. www.aavmc.org/data/files/vmcas/generalinfo.pdf

### Prerequisite Comparison Chart

A course requirement comparison chart of all AAVMC member schools. www.aavmc.org/data/files/vmcas/prerequisites.doc

### Test Chart

A showcase of the individual school test requirements and deadlines. www.aavmc.org/applicant-responsibilities/requirements.aspx (Scroll down to "test scores.")

### Fee Structure

VMCAS fees broken down by number of designations. www.aavmc.org/Applicant-Responsibilities/Fees.aspx

### Evaluation Requirements

Individual recommendation requirements by school. www.aavmc.org/Applicant-Responsibilities/Evaluations.aspx

### Supplemental Applications

Additional applications required by some schools. www.aavmc.org/supplemental.aspx

## VMCAS

1101 Vermont Ave NW Suite 301
Washington, DC 20005
Telephone: (617) 612-2884
Fax: (617) 612-2051
vmcasinfo@vmcas.org
www.aavmc.org

*S.E.T. stands for:
Submission: Have your application E-Submitted and Paid
Evaluations: Get at least one of your three evaluations submitted
Transcripts: Have all of your transcripts sent to and received by VMCAS

# VETERINARY MEDICAL SCHOOLS IN THE **UNITED STATES**

*AVMA/COE Accredited*

# AUBURN UNIVERSITY

Email Address: storyka@auburn.edu
Website: http://www.vetmed.auburn.edu

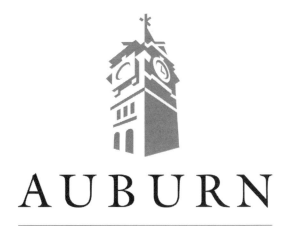

## SCHOOL DESCRIPTION

At Auburn, students have the opportunity to work in a collaborative environment with more than 100 nationally and internatinally recognized faculty to pursue needed answers to current challenges in areas such as biotechnology, oncology,criticl, genetics, infectious diseases, molecular medicine, neuroscience, gene therapy and nanotechnology.

> Students have the
> opportunity to
> work with more
> than 100 nationally
> and internatinally
> recognized faculty.

## APPLICATION INFORMATION

Full participant in VMCAS.

## SUMMARY OF ADMISSION PROCEDURES

*Application deadline:* October 2

*GRE score deadline:* October 2

*Notification of interview:* January-February

*Date interviews are held:* February-March

*Date acceptance notifications sent:* March

*Applicant's response date:* April 15

*Freshman orientation (mandatory):* August 5

*Regular classes begin:* August 11

*Deposit (to hold place in class):* none required

*Deferments:* not considered

*Transfer Students:* no

*International Students:* no

*Evaluation criteria:* Auburn University has a three part admission procedure, which entails an objective evaluation (academic credentials), a subjective review (personal credentials & work experience with animals), and a personal interview.

*Letters of Recommendation:* Three electronic evaluations are required, one from a veterinarian, one from an employer who might be a 2nd veterinarian and the third should be from an academician (major professor or advisor).

*Transcripts:* Transcripts are no longer mailed to the College of Veterinary Medicine.

*GRE Code:* 1005

Register early to get your preferred test date and location.

GRE Website

## ENTRANCE REQUIREMENTS

Alabama and Contract students must have a minimum cumulative gpa of 2.50 to be considered for admission. At-large applicants must hve a 3.90 cumulative gpa for consideration.

*Is a Bachelor's Degree Required?* no

*Is this an International School?* no

## ESTIMATED TUITION

*Estimated Tuition Resident:* $17,858

*Estimated Tuition Contract:* $17,858

*Estimated Tuition Non-Resident:* $42,382

## AVAILABLE SEATS

*Resident:* 40

*Contract:* 38

*Non-Resident:* 40

## TEST REQUIREMENTS

General GRE, verbal, quantitative and writing score

*VMCAS Participation:* full

*Accepts International Students?* no

## ADDITIONAL INFORMATION

*Application Deadline:* 10/2/2014

# UNIVERSITY OF CALIFORNIA

Email Address: admissions@vetmed.ucdavis.edu
Website: http://www.vetmed.ucdavis.edu

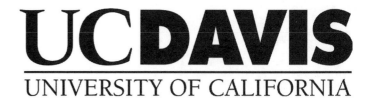

## SCHOOL DESCRIPTION

The University of California, Davis (UC Davis) campus is one of 10 campuses of the University of California system. It is the largest campus, with 5,200 acres. The Davis campus is located in Yolo County in the Central Valley of northern California. Davis is situated 11 miles west of Sacramento, 385 miles north of Los Angeles, and 72 miles northeast of San Francisco. Davis is surrounded by open space, including some of the most productive agricultural land in the state. The terrain is flat and the City of Davis is a friendly college town that cares about sustainability and welcoming newcomers. Ranked as one of the best towns to live in in the nation, Davis is also considered the most bike-friendly city in the nation. The Central Valley climate can be described as Mediterranean. The mild temperate climate means enjoyment of outdoors all year long. During the hot, dry, sunny summers, temperatures on some days can exceed 100 degrees F; however, more often summer temperatures are in the low 90s. Spring and fall has some of the most pleasant weather in the state. Winters in Davis are usually mild. UC Davis is an outstanding research and training institution with over 34,000 undergraduate, graduate and professional students. The Davis campus has four undergraduate colleges, graduate studies in all schools and colleges, and six professional programs carried out in the schools of Education, Law, Management, Medicine, Nursing, and Veterinary Medicine.

> UC Davis is an outstanding research and training institution with over 34,000 students.

Since 1948 the School of Veterinary Medicine serves the people of California by providing educational, research, clinical service, and public service programs of the highest quality to advance the health and care of animals, the health of the environment, and public health, and to contribute to the economy. School of Veterinary Medicine faculty members have earned a reputation for their broad expertise and shared commitment to solving some of society's most persistent health problems. The school's impact is evident in the accomplishments of clinicians who have developed novel treatments and basic scientists who continue to make major discoveries in animal, human and environmental health. We address the health of all animals, including livestock, poultry, companion animals, captive and free-ranging wildlife, exotic animals, birds, aquatic mammals and fish, and animals used in biological and medical research. Our expertise also encompasses related human health concerns.

To carry out this mission, we focus on students of our professional Doctor of Veterinary Medicine program, Master of Preventive Veterinary Medicine program, graduate clinical residency program and graduate academic MS and PhD programs. The school is fully committed to recruiting students with diverse backgrounds.

The School of Veterinary Medicine is home of the William R. Pritchard Veterinary Medical Teaching Hospital, Veterinary Medicine Teaching and Research Center, California Animal Health and Food Safety Laboratory, UC Veterinary Medical Center-San Diego and Centers of Excellence-fostering research, teaching and service focused on species interests and multidisciplinary themes. There are many other centers and innovative programs at UC Davis. Our statewide mission includes 28 research and clinical programs including continuing education; extension; and community outreach.

## PREREQUISITES FOR ADMISSION

| Course Description | Number of Hours/Credits | Necessity |
|---|---|---|
| General chemistry (with laboratory) | Two semesters (3 quarters) w/lab | Required |
| Organic chemistry (with laboratory) | Two semesters (2-3 quarters) w/lab | Required |
| Physics | Two semesters (2-3 quarters) | Required |
| General biology (with laboratory) | Two semesters (3 quarters) w/lab | Required |
| *Systemic physiology | One semester/quarter | Required |
| *Biochemistry (bioenergetics and metabolism) | One semester/quarter | Required |
| *Genetics (genes and gene expression) | One semester/quarter | Required |
| English composition and additional English | Two semesters | Required |
| Humanities and social sciences | Two semesters | Required |
| Statistics | One semester | Required |

*courses must be taken at the upper division level

## APPLICATION INFORMATION

For specific application information (availability, deadlines, fees, and VMCAS participation), please refer to our website at www.vetmed.ucdavis.edu.

*Residency implications:* A non-specified number of resident, nonresident, and WICHE applicants are accepted. International students are also considered for admission.

## SUMMARY OF ADMISSION PROCEDURES

*VMCAS application deadline:* Thursday, October 2, 2014 10:00 AM Pacific Standard Time

Supplemental information is required. School will notify applicant via portal after Oct. 2 deadline.

*Date interviews are held:* mid-December

*Date notifications available via portal:* mid-January

*School begins:* August

*Deposit (to hold place in class):* required

*Deferments:* only on case by case basis

## EVALUATION CRITERIA

Grades - Science GPA and Last 45 units

GRE Quantitative scores

PPI Evaluations (Three ETS PPI evaluations must be received by UC Davis no later than Oct. 2, 2014. PPI evaluations are in addition to the e-LORs required by VMCAS.)

MMI Interview

## ENTRANCE REQUIREMENTS

*Required undergraduate GPA:* a minimum grade point average of 2.50 on a 4.00 scale is required for all science courses completed and 2.50 on all courses cumulatively at time of application. Applicants admitted in fall 2013 had a mean cumulative GPA of 3.70.

*Is a Bachelor's Degree Required?* yes

*Is this an International School?* no

## ESTIMATED TUITION

*Estimated Tuition Resident:* $34, 213

*Estimated Tuition Contract:* $46,458

*Estimated Tuition Non-Resident:* $46,458

## AVAILABLE SEATS - 138

*Resident:* varied

*Contract:* varied

*Non-Resident:* varied

## TEST REQUIREMENTS

*Standardized examinations:* Graduate Record Examination, general test is required. The acceptable GRE test dates for applicants entering fall 2015 are September 1, 2009 - September 1, 2014. (Test code for UC Davis SVM is 4804.)

*VMCAS Participation:* full

*Accepts International Students?* yes

## ADDITIONAL INFORMATION

*Dual-Degree programs*

Combined DVM/PhD graduate degree programs are available.

Visit our Veterinary Scientist Training Program information at www.vetmed.ucdavis.edu/vstp.

*Application Deadline:* 10/2/2014

# COLORADO STATE UNIVERSITY

Email Address: dvmadmissions@colostate.edu
Website: http://csu-cvmbs.colostate.edu/
dvm-program/Pages/DVM-Program-Entrance-
Requirements.aspx

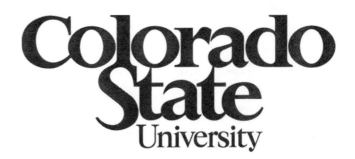

## SCHOOL DESCRIPTION

Colorado State University is located in Fort Collins, a city of about 150,000 in the eastern foothills of the Rocky Mountains about 65 miles north of Denver. Fort Collins has a pleasant climate and offers many cultural and recreational activities. Many of the state's ski areas lie within a short driving distance, making some of the best skiing in the world accessible. The nearby river canyons and mountain parks are beautiful scenic attractions and provide opportunities for hiking, fishing, photography, camping, and biking.

> Colorado State University is located in Fort Collins, a city of about 150,000 in the eastern foothills of the Rockies.

The College of Veterinary Medicine and Biomedical Sciences is nationally renowned for its programs in oncology, equine surgery and reproduction, and pain management. Our college is composed of eight major buildings that house the departments of biomedical sciences, environmental and radiological health sciences, and microbiology, immunology, and pathology.

The James L. Voss Veterinary Teaching Hospital, one of the world's largest and best equipped, houses the clinical sciences department. This department boasts a variety of unique units, including the internationally acclaimed Robert H. and Mary G. Flint Animal Cancer Center, Animal Population Health Institute, Integrated Livestock Management Program, and Gail Holmes Equine Orthopaedic Research Center. The hospital attracts a large caseload and offers students a wide variety of clinical experiences.

The uniquely designed Diagnostic Medicine Center houses the college's Veterinary Diagnostic Laboratory (VDL), the University's Extension Veterinarian, the Clinical Pathology Laboratory and the Animal Population Health Institute.

The VDL provides disease testing services to veterinarians, state/ federal agencies, livestock owners and pet owners. The Clinical Pathology Laboratory provides services such as blood, fluid and urine analysis and cytology to identify diseases and illnesses in animals brought to the VTH or to veterinarians in the region. The Animal Population Health Institute encourages collaboration and information and expertise exchange in veterinary epidemiology among scientists at CSU, collaborating institutions and government agencies throughout the world.

Internationally known for its innovative curriculum, our veterinary program provides students with a four-year course of study in veterinary medicine leading to the Doctor of Veterinary Medicine degree. The first two years are conducted on the main campus and include comprehensive coverage of veterinary and biomedical sciences along with integrated hands-on and clinical experiences. During the second two years, students participate in animal care at the Veterinary Teaching Hospital through a series of specialty rotations. Students participate as team members in evaluating patients, meeting with clients, developing treatment plans, and providing hands-on care, all under the supervision of faculty clinicians.

## PREREQUISITES FOR ADMISSION

| Course Description | Number of Semester/Credits | Necessity |
|---|---|---|
| Biochemistry (that requires Org Chem) | 3 | Required |
| Genetics | 3 | Required |
| Physics (with a laboratory) | 4 | Required |
| Statistics | 3 | Required |
| Lab associated with a biology course | 1 | Required |
| Lab associated with a chemistry course | 1 | Required |
| English Composition | 3 | Required |
| Social sciences and humanities | 12 | Required |
| Electives | 30 | Required |

## APPLICATION INFORMATION

*Application requirements:* The Colorado Supplemental Application is required. For your application to be reviewed by the Veterinary Admissions Committee, we must receive the following items before the deadline:

- VMCAS Application
- Colorado Supplemental Application and Fee
- GRE Verbal and Quantitative (self-reported/unofficial) scores

## SUMMARY OF ADMISSION PROCEDURES

*Colorado Supplemental Application deadline:* Thursday, October 2, 2014 at 11:00 AM (MT).

*VMCAS Application deadline:* Thursday, October 2, 2014 at 1:00 PM (ET).

*School begins:* late August

*Deposit:* (to hold place in class) none required

*Deferments:* case by case basis for extenuating circumstances

## EVALUATION CRITERIA

Quality of academic program (course load, challenging curriculum, honors)
GRE scores
Veterinary/Animal/Research/Work experience
Extracurricular/Community activities, achievements, leadership
Essay
Contribution to diversity, unique attributes, extenuating circumstances

Letters of Reference, pls see #6 at: http://csu-cvmbs.colostate.edu/dvm-program/Pages/DVM-Program-Entrance-Requirements.aspx

## ENTRANCE REQUIREMENTS

*Required undergraduate GPA:* No minimum requirement

*Mean GPA:* for the 2013 matriculated class was 3.60 on a 4.00 scale

*AP credits:* must appear on official transcript

*Course completion deadline:* transcript and final grades, including all required courses, must be received by JULY 15 prior to matriculation

*Is a Bachelor's Degree Required?* no

*Is this an International School?* no

## ESTIMATED TUITION

*Estimated Tuition Resident:* $26,451

*Estimated Tuition Contract:* $26,451

*Estimated Tuition Non-Resident:* $54,269

## AVAILABLE SEATS

*Resident:* 75

*Contract:* 30-35

*Non-Resident:* 30-35

## TEST REQUIREMENTS

The GRE General Test (Verbal and Quantitative) is required. The mean GRE scores for the 2013 matriculated class are Verbal 537/155 and Quantitative 664/150.

Test scores dated earlier than September 1, 2009, will not be accepted. It is the applicant's responsibility to schedule the test on or before September 30, 2014 so s/he can self-report unofficial scores on the Colorado Supplemental Application before the October 2, 2014 11:00am MT deadline. You will know your unofficial scores before leaving the testing center. NOTE: The self-reported unofficial Verbal and Quantitative scores must be entered into the Colorado Supplemental Application in order to submit the application.

*Sending official scores:* Applicants should submit a request to their testing center, before October 2, to have official scores sent to CSU (code 4075 and dept 0617). Scores should be received at CSU by November 30. In December, official scores will be used to verify all applicant self-reported scores before offers are made.

*VMCAS Participation:* full

*Accepts International Students?* yes

## ADDITIONAL INFORMATION

The veterinary program at CSU offers the following programs:

UAF (Alaska)/CSU: http://csu-cvmbs.colostate\.edu/dvm-program/Pages/uaf-csu-collaborative-veterinary-program.aspx

MBA/DVM: http://csu-cvmbs.colostate.edu/dvm-program/Pages/DVM-MBA.aspx

MPH/DVM: http://csu-cvmbs.colostate.edu/dvm-program/Pages/DVM-MPH.aspx

MST/DVM: http://csu-cvmbs.colostate.edu/dvm-program/Pages/DVM-MST.aspx

PhD/DVM: http://csu-cvmbs.colostate.edu/dvm-program/Pages/DVM-PhD.aspx

FAVCIP (Food Animal):

http://csu-cvmbs.colostate.edu/dvm-program/Pages/DVM-Special-Programs.aspx

*Application Deadline:* 10/2/2014

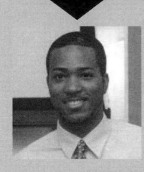

### Why do you want to be a veterinarian?

Since childhood, I have always respected the dynamic bond that people share with animals. The veterinarian plays a pivotal role in this relationship by maximizing its potentials and ensuring its longevity. Within the field of veterinary medicine, I have developed a strong interest in the conservation of endangered species and have aspirations of becoming a zoo and exotic animal veterinarian. Ultimately, I hope to help preserve our world's most beautiful and iconic creatures to ensure that they can continue to educate future generations about the important roles that they play.

### What are your short-term and long-term goals?

Currently, my short-term goals include gaining varied experience not only in exotics, but also in small and large animal medicine. I thoroughly believe that one interested in the field of zoo and exotic animal medicine should be comfortable and clinically proficient in domestic animal medical care. On a long-term basis, I plan to participate in a one-year post-doctoral internship in zoological medicine. After completion of this internship, I hope to finish a three-year residency in the field to become a diplomate of the American College of Zoological Medicine. Ultimately, I see myself working as a veterinarian at a zoological park and overseeing the healthcare of the park's collection.

### What did you do as an applicant to prepare for veterinary school?

My preparation in applying to veterinary school started when I was a freshman in high school enrolled in the math/science magnet program. In this program, I was exposed to many advanced courses in science related fields that challenged me to think independently and integrate knowledge on a more accelerated level. I also participated in various clubs and organizations, such as the Medical Sciences Club, which exposed students to various career options available in medicine. My senior year in high school, I was accepted to Tuskegee University, where I earned my degree in animal, poultry, and veterinary sciences. While at Tuskegee, I made sure to participate in the Pre-Vet Club as well as the Veterinary Scholar's Program, both of which exposed me to the field of veterinary medicine and allowed me to gain hands-on experience in animal care. During my summers as an undergraduate student, I was able to participate in two research programs at Kansas State University through the College of Agriculture. These internships gave me an opportunity to see not only how veterinary research is conducted, but also how the results of the study are interpreted and applied. Most importantly, outside of internships and volunteering in clinics, I put most emphasis on maintaining a competitive grade point average. This undeniably helped me in the application process and also facilitated my transition from undergraduate study to the curriculum of professional school.

### What advice would you give to applicants or those considering veterinary school?

My advice to applicants considering veterinary school is to stay focused and committed to your goal. While in high school, try to take as many advanced placement and honors classes as possible. The level of instruction in these classes mirrors that of college classes. In college, choose a major that will give both a solid foundation in the sciences and meet the course requirements for the veterinary schools being applied to. These would include animal sciences, biology, chemistry, and so forth. In college, it's best to get involved in extracurricular activities to be balanced and well-rounded. When applying to veterinary school, choose the individuals that will represent you through letters of recommendations wisely, for they will be the ones to attest to your work ethic, character, and integrity. Lastly, I would recommend getting all application materials checked by someone else to ensure that all requirements have been met.

### What is your advice on financial aid?

Primarily, entering the field of veterinary medicine is a responsibility that involves a significant amount of monetary dedication. When applying to veterinary school, research the schools of interest and pay particular attention to the rate of tuition. The cost of each veterinary school varies depending on different factors such as location, size, and state funding. However, there is a difference when comparing in-state and out-of-state tuition prices. In-state tuition prices are usually lower and are less taxing on the student's amount of debt. Possible sources of financial aid include scholarships by the university, federal student loans, and loans through banks. When applying for aid, ask questions and get a solid understanding of the loan, when funds will be provided to you, and the process of loan repayment.

# CORNELL UNIVERSITY

Email Address: vet_admissions@cornell.edu
Website: http://www.vet.cornell.edu/admissions

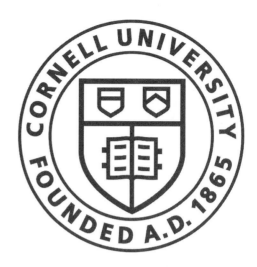

## SCHOOL DESCRIPTION

Cornell is located in Ithaca, a college town of about 30,000 in the Finger Lakes region of upstate New York, a beautiful area of rolling hills, deep valleys, scenic gorges, and clear lakes. The university's 740-acre campus is bounded on two sides by gorges and waterfalls. Open countryside, state parks, and year-round opportunities for outdoor recreation, including excellent sailing, swimming, skiing, hiking, and other activities, are only minutes away.

> The curriculum is interdisciplinary and focuses on the student as the primary force in learning.

Ithaca is one hour by air and a four-hour drive from New York City, and other major metropolitan areas are easily accessible. Direct commercial flights connect Ithaca with New York, Boston, Chicago, Pittsburgh, Philadelphia, and other cities.

The tradition of academic excellence, the cultural vigor of a distinguished university, and the magnificent setting create a stimulating environment for graduate study. The curriculum differs from other programs in that it is interdisciplinary, small group learning early in the program and focuses on the student as the primary force in learning.

## APPLICATION INFORMATION

For specific information about the application process visit our web site at: http://www.vet.cornell.edu/admissions/

The Supplemental Application can be found at: http://www.vet.cornell.edu/admissions/applicants/CornellSupplementalApplication.cfm

You may also subscribe to our free electronic Pre-Vet Newsletter at: http://www.vet.cornell.edu/admissions/PreVetNewsletters.cfm for application updates and current information about the College of Veterinary Medicine.

*Residency implications:* approximately 55 seats for New York State residents and 47 seats for non-NY residents

## SUMMARY OF ADMISSION PROCEDURES

*VMCAS application deadline:* Thursday, October 2, 2014 at 1:00 PM Eastern Time (transcripts due September 2, 2014, to VMCAS)

*Supplemental application deadline:* October 15

*Information sessions at the college for admitted students and alternates:* February/March

*Date acceptances mailed:* January

*School begins:* mid/late August

*Deposit (to hold place in class):* $500.00 (by April 15)

*Deferments:* considered on an individual basis, and ordinarily granted for illness or other situations beyond the control of the applicant.

## PREREQUISITES FOR ADMISSION

| Course Description | Number of Hours/Credits | Necessity |
| --- | :---: | :---: |
| English composition/literature* (full year) | 6 | Required |
| Biology or zoology, full year with laboratory | 6 | Required |
| Physics, full year with laboratory | 6 | Required |
| Inorganic (general) chemistry, full year with laboratory | 6 | Required |
| Organic chemistry, full year with laboratory | 6 | Required |
| Biochemistry, half year required; full year preferred | 4 | Required |
| General microbiology, with laboratory | 3 | Required |
| Non-prerequisite elective credits needed | 53 | Required |

*3 credits of literature may be satisfied by a course in public speaking

## EVALUATION CRITERIA

The following admissions formula allows the applicant to see how their application will be reviewed:

25% Overall GPA

25% GRE (verbal & quantitative) or MCAT Scores

20% Animal/Veterinary/Biomedical Research Experiences

• at least one letter of evaluation from a veterinarian

5% Quality of Academic Program

• with academic letter of evaluation

10% Non-Cognitive Skills

10% All Other Achievements

5% Personal Statement

## ENTRANCE REQUIREMENTS

*Required undergraduate GPA:* No specific GPA requirement, but the grade range of those admitted tends to be 3.00-4.00.

*AP credit policy:* accepted for physics and general or inorganic chemistry with a score of 4 or higher.

*Course completion deadline:* all but 12 credits of the prerequisite coursework should be completed at the time of application, with at least one semester of any two-semester series underway. Any outstanding prerequisites must be completed by the end of the spring term prior to matriculation.

*Is a Bachelor's Degree Required?* no

*Is this an International School?* no

## ESTIMATED TUITION

*Estimated Tuition Resident:* $30,725

*Estimated Tuition Contract:* n/a

*Estimated Tuition Non-Resident:* $45,575

## AVAILABLE SEATS

*Resident:* 55

*Contract:* 0

*Non-Resident:* 47

## TEST REQUIREMENTS

*Standardized examinations:* Graduate Record Examination (GRE), general test (verbal and quantitative), or the Medical College Admission Test (MCAT) is required. Official test scores must be received directly from ETS or AAMC by October 15th. Test scores older than five years will not be accepted.

*VMCAS Participation:* full

*Accepts International Students?* yes

## ADDITIONAL INFORMATION

*Combined Degree Programs*

*Combined DVM/PhD Program:* By integrating Cornell's veterinary and graduate curricula in the DVM/PhD Program, we prepare students to become leaders in science, medicine, and society, able to excel in basic research, cutting-edge medicine, and teaching. Students receive substantial financial funding incentives to complete both degrees.

*DVM/MPH (Masters in Public Health):* A partnership between the College of Veterinary Medicine and the University of Minnesota School of Public Health allows students the opportunity to earn a Master of Public Health (MPH) degree while completing their DVM training.

*For more information on both combined degree programs visit:* http://www.vet.cornell.edu/admissions/OADual Degree.cfm

*Other Admissions Programs*

*Sophomore Early Acceptance Program:* The Early Acceptance Program gives exceptionally well qualified applicants the opportunity to obtain admission to veterinary school after the completion of the sophomore year. With admission to the Cornell University College of Veterinary Medicine secured, the successful applicant may use the time between acceptance and matriculation to pursue experience in areas of personal interest. More information can be found at: http://www.vet.cornell.edu/admissions/applicants/OAEarlyAcceptance.cfm

*Transfer Student Admissions:* Cornell will consider applications for advanced standing in the DVM program on an individual basis, if an opening exists in the second-year class. More information can be found at: http://www.vet.cornell.edu/admissions/transfer_students.cfm

*Summer Research Opportunities*

*The Leadership Program for Veterinary Scholars:* A unique summer learning experience for veterinary students who seek to broadly influence the veterinary profession through a career in research. The program in an intensive research-oriented learning experience that combines faculty-guided research with career counseling, student-directed learning, and a variety of professional enrichment activities.

*Additional Summer Research Opportunities:* Additional summer research opportunities for veterinary students include the Veterinary Investigator Program, Veterinary Training in Biomedical Research, Aquavet, Summer Dairy Institute, the Food Animal Medicine Externship, and the Havemeyer Foundation Equine Research Fellowships.

*For more information about all of these summer research opportunities visit:* http://www.vet.cornell.edu/BBS/Scientists/SummerResearch.cfm

*Application Deadline:* 10/2/2014

# FIRST-YEAR PROFILE: COURTNEY HUNTER

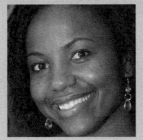

### Why do you want to be a veterinarian?
Like most veterinarians, I love animals. I always have since I was a little girl. The older I got, I realized that I also love science and have always been intrigued with medicine. I want to be a veterinarian because it is the only profession where I can be around animals every day and be challenged with scientific problems.

### What are your short-term and long-term goals?
I am a first-year vet student, so my short-term goal is to do the best I can in vet school and learn the most I can. In the long term, I hope to one day become a boarded laboratory animal veterinarian and receive my PhD.

### What did you do as an applicant to prepare for veterinary school?
I started the process of preparing for vet school pretty early. I became a volunteer at my city's zoo when I was twelve, and I stayed there throughout high school. I also worked at a local clinic in high school. In college I realized I was interested in research, so I contacted my state's vet school for summer research opportunities. For two summers I worked on a research project set up by a faculty member at the vet school and shadowed various areas in the animal hospital. After college, I took a year to finish my prerequisites and to do an internship at a sea turtle hospital in North Carolina so that I could get experience with aquatic medicine, another area I had an interest in.

### What advice would you give to applicants or those considering veterinary school?
I would tell applicants to first make sure they want to actually be a veterinarian. The best way I can think of to do this is to get lots of shadowing experience. Paid experience is great, but if a paid position is unavailable, I always found that most veterinarians were more than happy to let students shadow them multiple times. I would also say to shadow various types of veterinarians, not just the dog and cat vets most people think of. There are numerous areas in this field, and you never know what may spark an interest.

### What helped make the transition to veterinary school easier?
I was fortunate to meet a lot of students in the classes ahead of me before I entered vet school. Talking to them about what to expect helped me be prepared. I would encourage applicants to reach out to current vet students. We are busy, but I think most people would not mind taking time to answer a few questions about their experiences. We all probably had the same questions when we were applicants.

### What is your advice on financial aid?
Vet school is an investment, that is for sure. I have always been told to take out the very least amount in loans that I can and still survive on. There are scholarships available, but they may be hard to come by. That being said, I would apply for every scholarship I possibly could. You should also be smart with your loan money. The money is for school and living, not to splurge on unnecessary expenses.

### What are you most excited about learning in veterinary school?
I am in a dual degree DVM/PhD program where I started work on my graduate studies before vet school. I am excited to learn the medicine side behind my research. I study equine respiratory disease, so learning physiology and anatomy has been exciting for me so far. I am also excited to learn about disease next year and what exactly happens to the body as a result of various diseases.

### What advice do you have for students who are considering applying to veterinary school?
As a child I always knew that I wanted to be a veterinarian; however, I officially made the decision that I wanted to go to veterinary school in the ninth grade after a visit to the open house that Mississippi State University's College of Veterinary Medicine held annually. After I saw the animal hospital, heard the vet students give presentations, and talked to some of the clinicians, I knew that I wanted to be those people one day.

# UNIVERSITY OF FLORIDA

Email Address: studentservices@vetmed.ufl.edu
Website: http://www.vetmed.ufl.edu

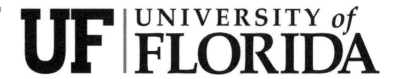

## SCHOOL DESCRIPTION

The University of Florida is located in Gainesville, a college town of approximately 125,000 in north central Florida, midway between the Gulf of Mexico and the Atlantic Ocean. Changes in season are marked, but winters are mild and permit year-round participation in outdoor activities.

The university accommodates about 50,000+ students with programs in almost all disciplines. The College of Veterinary Medicine is a component of the Institute of Food and Agricultural Sciences (which also includes Agriculture and Forest Resources and Conservation). It is also one of 6 colleges affiliated with the Health Science Center (the other 5 are Dentistry, Public Health and Health Professions, Medicine, Nursing, and Pharmacy).

> The veterinary curriculum is a 9-semester program consisting of core curriculum and elective experiences.

The veterinary curriculum is a 9-semester program consisting of core curriculum and elective experiences. The core provides the body of knowledge and skills common to all veterinarians. The first 4 semesters concentrate primarily on basic medical sciences. Students are additionally introduced to physical diagnosis, radiology, and clinical problems during these years. The core also includes experience in each of the clinical areas. Elective areas of concentration permit students to investigate further the aspects of both basic and clinical sciences most relevant to their interests.

## APPLICATION INFORMATION

For specific application information (availability, deadlines, fees, and VMCAS participation), please refer to the contact information listed above.

*Residency implications:* Florida has no contractual agreements. The college admits 88 Florida residents and 24 non-sponsored applicants each academic year. International applicants are included in the non-sponsored pool.

## SUMMARY OF ADMISSION PROCEDURES

*VMCAS application deadline:* Thursday, October 2, 2014 at 1:00 PM Eastern Time

*UF Professional School Application deadline:* September 1, 2014. Information on our supplemental requirements can be found at: www.vetmed.ufl.edu

*Date interviews are held:* February

*Date acceptances mailed:* March

*School begins:* mid-August

*Deposit (to hold place in class):* none required

*Deferments:* considered on an individual basis

## EVALUATION CRITERIA

The admission procedure consists of 3 parts: each applicant's file is reviewed; selected applicants are each interviewed for about 1 hour by 3 admissions committee panel; final selection of new class takes place.

| Course Description | Number of Hours/Credits | Necessity |
| --- | --- | --- |
| Biology (general, genetics, microbiology) | 15 | Required |
| Chemistry (inorganic, organic, biochemistry) | 19 | Required |
| Physics | 8 | Required |
| Mathematics (calculus, statistics) | 6 | Required |
| Animal Science (introduction to animal science, animal nutrition) | 6 | Required |
| Humanities | 9 | Required |
| Social sciences | 6 | Required |
| English (2 courses in English composition) | 6 | Required |
| Electives | 5 | Required |

## ENTRANCE REQUIREMENTS

*Suggested undergraduate GPA:* a minimum GPA of 3.0 on a 4.00 scale. The class of 2017 had an overall mean science prerequisite GPA of 3.56.

*Course completion deadline:* We encourage that 80% of the Science and Math pre-requisite courses (excluding Animal Sciences and Animal Nutrition) be completed by the end of the spring 2014 term to be included in the academic assessment.

*Is a Bachelor's Degree Required?* no

*Is this an International School?* no

## ESTIMATED TUITION

*Estimated Tuition Resident:* $28,630

*Estimated Tuition Contract:* $0

*Estimated Tuition Non-Resident:* $45,500

## AVAILABLE SEATS

*Resident:* 88

*Contract:* 0

*Non-Resident:* 24

## TEST REQUIREMENTS

*Standardized examinations:* Graduate Record Examination (GRE) is required. To be considered for Class of 2019 admissions cycle, the last day to sit for the GRE is September 1, 2014.

*VMCAS Participation:* full

*Accepts International Students?* yes

## ADDITIONAL INFORMATION

*Supplemental Application Deadline:* 9/1/2014

# UNIVERSITY OF GEORGIA

Email Address: dvmadmit@uga.edu

Website: http://www.vet.uga.edu/admissions

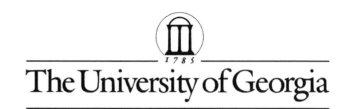

## SCHOOL DESCRIPTION

The University of Georgia is located in Athens-Clarke County, with a population of over 100,000. Georgia's Classic City is a prospering community that reflects the charm of the Old South while growing in culture and industry (www. visitathensga.com). Athens is just over an hour away from the north Georgia mountains and the metropolitan area of Atlanta, and just over 5 hours away from the Atlantic coast.

> The University of Georgia has grown into an institution with 16 schools and colleges and more than 2,889 faculty.

In 1785, Georgia became the first state to grant a charter for a state-supported university. In 1801 the first students came to the newly formed frontier town of Athens. The University of Georgia has grown into an institution with 16 schools and colleges and more than 2,889 faculty members and 34,519 students.

## APPLICATION INFORMATION

For specific application information (availability, deadlines, fees, and VMCAS participation), please refer to the contact information listed above.

Residency implications: Georgia retains up to 19 positions for contract students. Contracts are with Delaware (maximum 2 seats) and South Carolina (maximum 17 seats). The balance of those admitted are residents of Georgia or nonresident, non-contract applicants. International applications are accepted. Total number of students admitted each year: 114.

*Residency implications:* Anticipated class distribution is 40 Alabama residents, 38 Kentucky residents, 2 West Virginia residents and 40 non-contract non-resident students.

## SUMMARY OF ADMISSION PROCEDURES

*VMCAS application deadline:* October 2, 2014 1:00 PM Eastern Time

*Supplemental application deadline:* October 2, 2014 1:00 PM Eastern Time (The deadline to request a supplemental application account will be posted on our website).

*GRE score deadline:* October 2, 2014 (scores must be submitted electronically from ETS) (Applicant must use code 5752).

*Decision letters mailed:* late February

*School begins:* mid-August. A required 6-day orientation will precede the start of classes.

*Deposit (to hold place in class):* $500; $750 for nonresident, noncontract students.

*Deferments:* one-year deferments considered on a case-by-case basis.

## EVALUATION CRITERIA

The admissions procedure includes a file evaluation. There are no interviews.

## ADDITIONAL REQUIREMENTS AND CONSIDERATIONS

Program of Study
Animal/Veterinary Experience
References
Employment History
Personal Statement
Extracurricular Activities
Entrance Requirements

## PREREQUISITES FOR ADMISSION

| Course Description | Number of Hours/Credits | Necessity |
|---|---|---|
| English (writing intensive) | 6 | Required |
| Humanities and social studies | 14 | Required |
| General biology with lab (for science majors) | 8 | Required |
| Advanced biological science* | 8 | Required |
| Chemistry with lab - Inorganic | 8 | Required |
| Chemistry with lab - Organic | 8 | Required |
| Physics with lab | 8 | Required |
| Biochemistry (lab not required) | 3 | Required |

*Required undergraduate GPA:* cumulative GPA of 3.00 or greater on a 4.00 scale or a combined score on the GRE verbal and quantitative sections of 1200 on the old scale or 308 or higher on the new scale.

*Is a Bachelor's Degree Required?* no

*Is this an International School?* no

## ESTIMATED TUITION

*Estimated Tuition Resident:* approx. $18,000

*Estimated Tuition Contract:* approx. $18,000

*Estimated Tuition Non-Resident:* $44,320

## AVAILABLE SEATS

*Resident:* 80

*Contract:* 19

*Non-Resident:* 15

## TEST REQUIREMENTS

Standardized examinations: Graduate Record Examination (GRE) general test (including the analytical writing portion) must be completed within the 5 years immediately preceding the deadline for receipt

*VMCAS Participation:* full

*Accepts International Students?* yes

## ADDITIONAL INFORMATION

*Combined DVM-graduate degree programs are available:*

DVM-MPH Veterinarians in Public Health

DVM/PhD Veterinary Medical Scientist Training Program

*Application Deadline:* 10/2/2014

# UNIVERSITY OF ILLINOIS

Email Address: admissions@vetmed.illinois.edu
Website: http://vetmed.illinois.edu

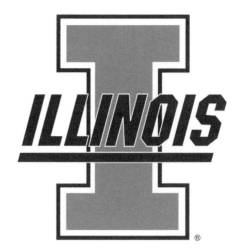

## SCHOOL DESCRIPTION

The University of Illinois is in Urbana-Champaign, a community of about 100,000 people located 140 miles south of Chicago. It is served by two airlines, 3 interstate highways, bus, and rail. The twin cities and university make a pleasant community with easy access to all areas and facilities. The university has about 42,000 students and more than 11,000 faculty and staff members. It is known for its high-quality academic programs and its exceptional resources and facilities. The university library has the largest collection of any public university and ranks third among all U.S. academic libraries. The university also has outstanding cultural and sports facilities and activities.

> It is known for its high-quality academic programs and its exceptional resources and facilities.

The College of Veterinary Medicine is located at the south edge of the campus. In addition to approximately 480 students, the college has about 100 graduate students plus a full complement of residents and interns. There are more than 100 full-time faculty with research interests in a variety of biomedical sciences and clinical areas. This research activity offers a broad variety of experiences for students. The college also offers students a dynamic, integrated core-elective curriculum to prepare for careers in almost any area of the profession.

## APPLICATION INFORMATION

For specific application information (availability, deadlines, fees, and VMCAS participation), please refer to our website: http://vetmed.illinois.edu/dvm-admissions

A Supplemental Application specific to the University of Illinois is required and may be obtained from the College Admissions website at: https://vetmed.illinois.edu/admissions/

International applications are considered, although there obvious constraints regarding translation of grades. The TOEFL will be required of any successful applicant before matriculation. U.S. Visa constraints may also be restrictive for admission.

*Residency implications:* priority is given to approximately 85 Illinois residents; approximately 35 nonresident positions are available.

## SUMMARY OF ADMISSION PROCEDURES

*VMCAS application deadline:* Thursday, October 2, 2014 at 1:00 PM Eastern Daylight Savings Time (noon Central Daylight Time)

*Informational program and required interviews:* Mid-February

*National application acceptance date:* April 15, 2015

*Date acceptances mailed:* late February-early March

*School begins:* late August

*Deposit (to hold place in class):* $500 deposit required on acceptance. Please check the Illinois Admissions website for the most current information.

## PREREQUISITES FOR ADMISSION

| Course Description | Number of Hours/Credits | Necessity |
| --- | --- | --- |
| Biological Science (with Lab) | 8 | Required |
| Chemical Sciences | 16 | Required |
| Physics w/ Lab | 8 | Required |
| English Composition | 3 | Required |
| Speech Communication | 3 | Required |
| Humanities / Social Science | 12 | Required |

*Deferments:* considered on an individual basis by the Associate Dean for Academic and Student Affairs.

## EVALUATION CRITERIA

A 3-part admission procedure is used. An academic evaluation and an application evaluation of veterinary, animal experience and personal qualities are followed by a personal interview.

*Academic evaluation:* GRE test scores; science GPA; cumulative GPA; rigor of academic preparation

*Nonacademic evaluation:* veterinary-related experience, animal-related experience, community involvement, leadership, citizenship, and letters of recommendation; interview

## ENTRANCE REQUIREMENTS

*Required undergraduate GPA:* a minimum cumulative GPA of 2.75 and a minimum science GPA of 2.75 on a 4.00 scale are required. The average statistics for students making it past Admissions Phase I in 2013 were 3.57 cumulative GPA, 3.44 science GPA, and 63% GRE composite percentile

*AP credit policy:* AP credit is allowed to meet the 8 s.h. physics prerequisite requirement if a student is awarded the full 8 s.h. AP credit is allowed for biology and chemistry if it is followed up by more advanced college-level courses in those science areas.

GRE test within two years of application. Refer to website for specific dates.

*Is a Bachelor's Degree Required?* no

*Is this an International School?* no

## ESTIMATED TUITION

*Estimated Tuition Resident:* $29,604

*Estimated Tuition Contract:* $0

*Estimated Tuition Non-Resident:* $47,068

## AVAILABLE SEATS

*Resident:* 85

*Contract:* 0

*Non-Resident:* 35

## TEST REQUIREMENTS

Standardized examinations: Graduate Record Examination (GRE), general test, is required. Test must be taken by September 15, 2014 for the 2014/2015 admission cycle (no test taken after September 15

*VMCAS Participation:* full

*Accepts International Students?* yes

## ADDITIONAL INFORMATION

Combined DVM/PhD programs may be available. DVM/MPH with concurrent enrollment at University of Illinois at Chicago, School of Public Health are also available.

DVM/PhD Veterinary Medical Scientist Training Program

*Application Deadline:* 10/2/2014

# IOWA STATE UNIVERSITY

Email Address: cvmadmissions@iastate.edu
Website: www.vetmed.iastate.edu

**IOWA STATE UNIVERSITY**
**College of Veterinary Medicine**

## SCHOOL DESCRIPTION

The Iowa State University College of Veterinary Medicine is located in the heart of one of the world's most intensive livestock-producing areas, which provides diverse food-animal clinical and diagnostic cases. A nearby metropolitan area and a regionally recognized referral veterinary hospital provide experience in companion-animal medicine and surgery. A strong basic science education during the first two years prepares veterinary students for a wide range of clinical experiences during the last two years. The College of Veterinary Medicine provides education in a wide variety of animal species and disciplines and allows fourth-year students to spend time with private practitioners, other colleges, research facilities, and in other educational experiences. Opportunities for research exist in the outstanding research programs in neurobiology, immunobiology, infectious diseases, and numerous other areas. The nearby National Animal Disease Center and the National Veterinary Services Laboratories provide additional research opportunities. The world's premier State Diagnostic Laboratory is part of the college and provides students with experience that is unmatched by any other veterinary college in the world. Graduates are highly sought after and can typically choose among five or six job offers. A career development and placement service is also provided.

> Iowa State University graduates are highly sought after and can typically choose among five or six job offers.

## APPLICATION INFORMATION

The most current application information (availability, deadlines, fees, VMCAS participation), may be found at: http://vetmed.iastate.edu/academics/prospective-students/admissions

*Supplemental Application:* A supplemental application is required. The supplemental becomes available June 1 and the link can be found at: http://vetmed.iastate.edu/academics/prospective-students/admissions

*Residency implications:* priority is given to Iowa residents for approximately 60 positions. Iowa contracts on a year-to-year basis with North Dakota, South Dakota and Connecticut. Iowa also has a formal educational alliance with Nebraska. Remaining positions are available for residents of noncontract states or international students.

## SUMMARY OF ADMISSIONS PROCEDURES

*Application deadline:* Iowa Residents: September 2, 2014

*All other applicants:* Tuesday, October 2, 2014 1:00 PM Eastern Time

*Date acceptances mailed:* Approximately February 15

*School begins:* late August

*Deposit (to hold place in class):* $500.00

*Deferments:* considered on a case-by-case basis

## EVALUATION CRITERIA

The admission procedure consists of a review of each candidate's application and qualifications:
1. Academic factors include grades, test scores, and courseload.

## PREREQUISITES FOR ADMISSION

| Course Description | Number of Hours/Credits | Necessity |
|---|---|---|
| General chemistry (1 year series w/lab) | 7 | Required |
| Organic chemistry (1 year series w/lab) | 7 | Required |
| Biochemistry | 3 | Required |
| Biology (1 year series w/labs) | 8 | Required |
| Genetics (Upper level Mendelian and molecular) | 3 | Required |
| Mammalian anatomy and/or physiology | 3 | Required |
| Oral communication | 3 | Required |
| (interpersonal, group or public speaking) | | |
| English composition | 6 | Required |
| Social Science/Humanities | 8 | Required |
| Physics | 4 | Required |
| (Physics 1 - first semester of a 2 semester series) | | |

2. Nonacademic factors include essays, experience, recommendations, and personal development activities.
3. Interviews are conducted.

## ENTRANCE REQUIREMENTS

*Required undergraduate GPA:* the minimum GPA required is 2.50 on a 4.00 scale. The most recent entering class had a mean GPA of 3.54.

*AP credit policy:* must be documented by original scores submitted to the university, and must meet the university's minimum requirement in the appropriate subject area. CLEP (College-Level Examination Program) credits accepted only for the arts, humanities, and social sciences.

*Course completion deadline:* It is preferred that prerequisite science courses be completed by the end of the fall term the year the applicant applies, and these must be completed with a C (2.0) or better to fulfill the requirement. However, up to 2 prerequisite science courses may be taken the spring term prior to matriculation. All other prerequisites must be completed by the end of the spring term prior to matriculation with a C (2.0) or better. Pending courses may not be completed the summer prior to matriculation. Pass-not pass grades are not acceptable.

*Is a Bachelor's Degree Required?* no

*Is this an International School?* no

## ESTIMATED TUITION

*Estimated Tuition Resident:* $20,014

*Estimated Tuition Contract:* Varies by contract

*Estimated Tuition Non-Resident:* $44,768

## AVAILABLE SEATS

*Resident:* 60

*Contract:* 41

*Non-Resident:* 48

## TEST REQUIREMENTS

*Standardized examinations:* Graduate Record Examination (GRE), general test, is required. Either the new Revised GRE or the previous GRE will be accepted but the scores must come directly from GRE.

*VMCAS Participation:* full

*Accepts International Students?* yes

# KANSAS STATE UNIVERSITY

Kansas State University
College of Veterinary Medicine
Email Address: admit@vet.k-state.edu
Website: http://www.vet.k-state.edu/

# KANSAS STATE
# UNIVERSITY

## SCHOOL DESCRIPTION

Kansas State University in Manhattan, Kansas, is located 125 miles west of Kansas City near Interstate 70. With a population of about 70,000 including KSU, Manhattan is in an area surrounded by many historical points of interest in a rich agricultural area of north central Kansas. Recreational activities abound in Manhattan and the surrounding area with fishing, boating, camping, and hunting among the favorites. Sporting events, theater, concerts, and excellent parks contribute to the many activities available. Kansans enjoy the 4 seasons, each of which brings its own special activities and events.

Kansas State University is on a beautiful 664-acre campus. The College of Veterinary Medicine opened in 1905. It is located on 80 acres just north of the main campus in 3 connected buildings.

> The College of Veterinary Medicine is located on 80 acres just north of the main campus in 3 connected buildings.

## APPLICATION INFORMATION

For specific application information (availability, deadlines, fees, and VMCAS participation), please refer to the contact information listed above.

*Supplemental Application:* Available at http://www. vet.k-state.edu/admit/apply.htm between June 1 and October 1.

*Contract tuition:* resident tuition

*Resident seats:* approximately 45

*Contract seats:* 5 with North Dakota

*Residency implications:* to be eligible to be in the Kansas pool of applicants, the applicant must be a Kansas resident for tuition purposes at the time of application. Kansas accepts about 60 nonresident students per year. International applicants are considered. Kansas has a contract for students from North Dakota.

## SUMMARY OF ADMISSION PROCEDURES

*Timetable*

*VMCAS application deadline:* October 2, 2014 at 1:00 PM Eastern Time

*Kansas State University supplemental application deadline:* postmarked by Wednesday, October 1, 2014

*Kansas residents:* mid-December

*Nonresident:* early January

*North Dakota:* February

*Date acceptances mailed:* within 6 weeks after interview

*School begins:* mid-August

*Deposit (to hold place in class):* $500.00

*Deferments:* may be considered by Admissions Committee for extraordinary circumstances.

## EVALUATION CRITERIA

A 4-part admission procedure is used, including evaluation of science grades, evaluation of all 3 GRE scores, assessment of the application and narrative, and a personal interview.

30%: Prerequisite science GPA

40%: Test scores

## PREREQUISITES FOR ADMISSION

| Course Description | Number of Hours/Credits | Necessity |
|---|---|---|
| Expository Writing I and II | 6 | Required |
| Public Speaking | 2 | Required |
| Chemistry I and II | 8 | Required |
| General Organic Chemistry w/lab | 5 | Required |
| General Biochemistry | 3 | Required |
| Physics I and II | 8 | Required |
| Principles of Biology or General Zoology | 4 | Required |
| Microbiology w/lab | 4 | Required |
| Genetics | 3 | Required |
| Social Sciences and/or Humanities | 12 | Required |
| Electives | 9 | Required |

30%: Interview score including:

References

Animal/veterinary experience

Leadership in college and community

Autobiographical essay

## ENTRANCE REQUIREMENTS

*Prerequisites for Admission:* Science courses must have been taken within six years of the date of enrollment in the professional program.

*Required undergraduate GPA:* the minimum required GPA to qualify for an interview is 2.80 on a 4.00 scale in both the prerequisite courses and the last 45 semester hours of undergraduate work. The most recent entering class had a mean prerequisite science GPA of 3.50.

*AP credit policy:* must appear on official college transcripts and be equivalent to the appropriate college-level coursework.

*Course completion deadline:* prerequisite courses must be completed by the end of the spring term of the year in which admission is sought.

*Standardized examinations:* Graduate Record Examination (GRE), general test, scores are required by October 1, unless all prerequisites are completed at Kansas State University.

## ADDITIONAL REQUIREMENTS AND CONSIDERATIONS

Animal/veterinary work experience and knowledge

Employment record

3 evaluations required by nonfamily members: one veterinarian, one academic or preprofessional advisor, one professor or other professional.

*Is a Bachelor's Degree Required?* no

*Is this an International School?* no

## ESTIMATED TUITION

*Estimated Tuition Resident:* $23,176.20

*Estimated Tuition Contract:* $23,176.20

*Estimated Tuition Non-Resident:* $50,463.60

## AVAILABLE SEATS

*Resident:* 45

*Contract:* 5

*Non-Resident:* about 60

## TEST REQUIREMENTS

Graduate Record Examination (GRE), general test

*VMCAS Participation:* full

*Accepts International Students?* yes

## ADDITIONAL INFORMATION

*Dual-Degree Programs*

Combined DVM-graduate degree programs are available.

Combined DVM-MPH degree programs are available.

*Early Admission Program*

The Veterinary Scholars Early Admission Program is designed for those students having a genuine desire to enter the veterinary profession who attend Kansas State University with an ACT score of 29 or greater or an equivalent SAT score and who complete a successful interview during the fall semester of their freshman undergraduate year.

*Application Deadline:* Thursday, October 2, 2014 at 1:00 PM Eastern Time

# FIRST-YEAR PROFILE: JULIANNA FRUM

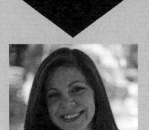

### Why do you want to be a veterinarian?

When I was very young, I always said I wanted to be a veterinarian. At some point in my teenage years, I decided to join the military instead. After attending undergrad on a US Navy ROTC scholarship at North Carolina State University, I was commissioned in the United States Navy. Although I was always proud to serve, I knew after my first year that this wasn't my calling. I began to work my way back into school to take classes so that I could fulfill my lifelong dream of being a veterinarian. The more experience I received, the more I realized that I wanted to serve my community as a small animal veterinarian. My own dog has needed emergency, life-saving care twice in the past three years, and I have experienced firsthand how valuable it is to have a local veterinarian who cares and does not know the meaning of "office hours" when an emergency strikes.

### What are your short-term and long-term goals?

My short-term goals are, of course, to continue being successful as a veterinary student. Mississippi State University's College of Veterinary Medicine has a unique curriculum that allows its students a lot of opportunities to experience the different aspects of veterinary medicine. Although I feel like small animal medicine is where my heart is, I don't want to rule out any other fields just yet. For a long-term goal, I just hope to be successful in whatever field of veterinary medicine I chose to focus on. I hope that I will be afforded the opportunity to participate in externships that may turn into employment opportunities as I close in on my graduation date.

### What did you do as an applicant to prepare for veterinary school?

I was fortunate enough to have amazing guidance from my academic advisors at West Virginia University. Dr. Margaret Minch took me under her wing and definitely helped me navigate returning to academia as an older, unconventional student. I met with Dr. Minch many times during the application process, as well in order to ensure that I was making the most of my application to veterinary school. I also spent years working as a veterinary tech and as a volunteer at local small animal hospitals to learn the ins and outs of the field. It was important to me to see the downside of the profession, to have to assist in euthanasia, and to be a part of those situations where you are unable to help the pet, to see if this was something I could emotionally handle. I believe that my many experiences have definitely helped to prepare me for my future.

### What advice would you give to applicants or those considering veterinary school?

No matter how difficult you think it will be, if being a veterinarian is what you want to do, then it is worth it. I would definitely recommend getting as much experience in as many different fields of veterinary medicine as you can manage. It will only help you in veterinary school to understand both small animal and large animal medicine.

### What helped make the transition to veterinary school easier?

Talking to my mentors who are fairly new veterinarians about how they viewed vet school helped me prepare for what to expect. Also, Mississippi State University's CVM has fantastic faculty who are constantly available to answer any questions we had prior to starting our first semester. We also have a Facebook group for the class of 2017 that really helped us interact with our peers prior to starting classes.

### What is your advice on financial aid?

Only take out what you calculate you need. Make a budget for yourself and do your very best to stick to it. Every penny that you borrow, you will be paying back and then some, so it will only help you to take out no more than you need every year.

### What are you most excited about learning in veterinary school?

I love learning about topics and breeds that I have very little experience with. I was able to participate in a slaughter lab for the American Association of Bovine Practitioners Student Club, and although it doesn't sound glamorous, it was extremely interesting to learn about some large animal practices that I have very little knowledge of.

# LINCOLN MEMORIAL UNIVERSITY

Email Address: veterinaryadmissions@lmunet.edu
Website: http://www.vetmed.lmunet.edu

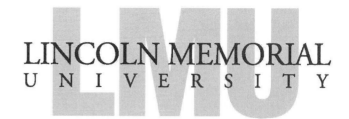

## SCHOOL DESCRIPTION

Lincoln Memorial University (LMU) is an accredited, independent, private, not-for-profit university founded through Abraham Lincoln's desire to organize a great university for the people of Appalachia. The campus is located in Harrogate, Tennessee, beautifully situated at the foot of historic Cumberland Gap, the 18th century gateway to the west pioneered by Daniel Boone. Only 58 miles north of Knoxville and 132 miles south of Lexington KY, LMU centrally located between two major cities that offer many cultural and recreational opportunities. The nearby Cumberland Gap National Historic Park is a favorite location for LMU students to hike, run, bicycle, and relax in between classes throughout the semester.

> Founded through Abraham Lincoln's desire to organize a great university for the people of Appalachia.

The LMU campus occupies more than 1,000 beautiful wooded acres, with modern educational facilities that include smart technology classrooms and laboratories. The University has a combined enrollment of 4300 undergraduate, graduate and professional students and awards the baccalaureate, master's and doctoral degrees. The University's professional programs include veterinary medicine, veterinary technology, nursing, physician's assistant, osteopathic medicine, law, medical laboratory science, and athletic training. Lincoln Memorial University's mission is three-fold: values-based service to humanity, providing educational and research op-portunities to students, and advancing life throughout the Appalachian region and beyond.

*Curriculum*

The College of Veterinary Medicine (CVM) curriculum is a four-year, 8 semester, program of study culminating in the Doctor of Veterinary Medicine (DVM) degree. The curriculum is based on the philosophy of clinical immersion as a practical approach to professional education that recognizes medical knowledge must be developed side-by-side with clinical skills. Clinical skills are developed in 3 areas of instructional emphasis: (1) veterinary problem-solving and clinical judgment, (2) client communication, and (3) technical proficiency in the performance of routine and advanced veterinary procedures. The overall aim of the clinical immersion curriculum is to maximize clinical competency of our students upon graduation. The pre-clinical sciences are taught on the LMU-CVM campus in semesters 1 through 5 as a foundation to developing an integrated understanding of the structure and interrelated function of the normal animal, and the mechanisms of disease. Course content is delivered via a modified approach to the study of body systems, in which the relevant structure (anatomy) and function (physiology) are presented together. This approach helps the student develop a comprehensive and practical understanding of the body's systems, and begins to train the mind in the discipline of clinical reasoning or "thinking like a doctor" essential for the clinical experiences that occur in semesters 6 through 8. The entire curriculum is taught with the One Health philosophy in mind. One Health recognizes the interaction between the health of animals, humans, and our shared environment, at both the individual and population levels.

## PREREQUISITES FOR ADMISSION

| Course Requirements[1] | Semester Hours | Quarter hours |
| --- | --- | --- |
| Biology (with laboratory) | 8 | 10 |
| Genetics | 3 | 4 |
| Biochemistry | 3 | 4 |
| Advanced Science Electives[2] | 8 | 10 |
| Organic Chemistry (with laboratory) | 6 | 8 |
| General Chemistry (with laboratory) | 8 | 10 |
| Physics | 3 | 4 |
| English | 6 | 8 |
| Probability and Statistics | 3 | 4 |
| Social and Behavioral Sciences[3] | 6 | 8 |
| Electives[4] | 6 | 8 |

1. Subject to change in the future
2. Upper division courses (300 level or higher) including Anatomy, Animal Science, Cell Biology, Immunology, Microbiology, Molecular Biology, Physiology, Virology
3. Potential courses include, but are not limited to: Anthropology, Economics, Geography, Philosophy, Political Science or Sociology. Also included: Ethics, Critical Thinking, Cultural Diversity, Social Responsibility, One Health, Human Animal Bond.
4. Potential courses include but are not limited to: Business, Communications, Foreign Language, History, and Public Speaking

*Clinical Experience*

The LMU-CVM recognizes the intensely practical nature of veterinary medicine and that the successful veterinarian must be able to integrate knowledge with a broad array of clinical and professional skills in order to successfully treat disease, prevent disease, and effectively communicate in a clinical setting. Therefore, as part of the clinical immersion concept, the CVM places a high emphasis on the development of clinical and professional skills throughout the curriculum.

The process begins at the LMU-CVM campus, where under the tutelage of the faculty, students will participate in structured laboratory sessions in order to develop diverse skills such as physical examination, diagnostic skills, surgical skills, therapeutic skills, how to work as both a member and leader of a health care team, and how to communicate effectively with clients and colleagues. This in-house phase of clinical experience begins in the first semester and builds throughout the pre-clinical courses. Beginning in the Fall term of the third year students receive a comprehensive review and refine their clinical and surgical skills in preparation for the distributed clinical portion of the curriculum.

During the clinical experience, students are sent to community based distributed clinical sites throughout the region and nation where they continue refining their knowledge, and professional and clinical skills. Each distributed clinical site has been carefully chosen by the CVM; and participating mentors are adjunct members of the CVM faculty. These highly experienced and dedicated veterinarians have a demonstrated commitment to excellence in teaching and in mentoring.

## APPLICATION INFORMATION

For specific information on applying to LMU College of Veterinary Medicine (availability, deadlines, fees and VMCAS participation) please refer to our website. LMU-CVM will admit 100 students for 2014-2015 admissions cycle.

*Residency implications:* Applicants from all states as well as international applicants will be considered. In-state and out-of-state applicants are given equal consideration.

## SUMMARY OF ADMISSION PROCEDURES

*Timetable*

*VMCAS application deadline:* Thursday, October 2, 2014, 1:00 PM Eastern Time

*Supplemental application and GRE score deadline:* Thursday, October 16, 2014, 1:00PM Eastern Time

Applications will not be considered by the Admissions Committee until the file is complete. Applications not completed by the October 16th deadline will be withdrawn from the application process.

*On-campus Interviews are held:* October to January

Students will be notified of the Admission Committee's decision within 3 weeks following the interview. Admission Committee decisions will be one of the following: Accept, Pending, or Deny.

In accordance with the Association of American Veterinary Medical Colleges acceptance deadline policy, students are not required to accept an offer of admission prior to April 15, 2015. The LMU-CVM deadline to submit matriculation paperwork and fee is April 15, 2015.

## EVALUATION CRITERIA

Applicants will be invited to campus for interviews based on holistic evaluation of their complete application with consideration to the following criteria:

Academic record

Overall GPA, Science GPA, GPA in last 2 years of full time study

GRE score

Non-technical skills/Aptitudes

Professional potential based on references and recommendations provided in the electronically submitted evaluations and letters of reference

Life experiences that demonstrate a balance of academic, work, community and personal commitments

Submission of a personal statement that (a) communicates knowledge of the veterinary profession, (b) summarizes personal experiences that have shaped the applicant's interest in veterinary medicine, including type(s) and amount of veterinary-related experience.

## ENTRANCE REQUIREMENTS

All pre-requisites course must be completed with grade of a C (2.0) or higher; C- grades will not be accepted.

All science pre-requisites must be completed within the last 10 years. Courses completed prior to August 2005 will not be considered.

*AP credit policy:* Must appear on official college transcripts and be equivalent to the appropriate college-level coursework.

*Required undergraduate GPA:* To be considered for admission, applicants must have a cumulative GPA of at least 2.8 on a 4.00 scale upon completion of a minimum of 50% of the credits required for a baccalaureate degree from a regionally accredited college or university.

Alternatively, students not meeting a GPA of <2.8, who have demonstrated a commitment to academic excellence (GPA >3.1) in the last 2 years of study (45 semester hours) may be considered on a case by case basis.

*Course completion deadline:* All prerequisite courses must be completed by the end of the spring term prior to matriculation. Final grades for all prerequisite courses must be verified prior to registration for LMU-CVM courses. Official transcripts must be submitted and verified by VMCAS directly following the completion of both Fall and Spring Semesters.

*Is a Bachelor's Degree Required?* no

*Is this an International School?* no

## ESTIMATED TUITION

*Estimated Tuition Resident:* $40,241.00 (subject to change)

*Estimated Tuition Contract:* 0

*Estimated Tuition Non-Resident:* $40,241.00

## AVAILABLE SEATS

*Resident:* pending

*Contract:* pending

*Non-Resident:* pending

## TEST REQUIREMENTS

The Graduate Record Examination (GRE) that includes verbal, quantitative, and analytic sub-sections is required for all applicants. The GRE scores must be current within the last 3 years of the application. The score code for LMU-CVM is 7576 (Lincoln Memorial Univ Vet Med). For applicants planning to matriculate in August 2015, results of GRE tests taken prior to August 2012 will not be accepted. Computer-based GRE tests must be taken by September 30, 2014 in order for

LMU-CVM to receive the scores by the October 16th deadline. We encourage you to take the test well in advance of the deadline.

The Test of English as a Foreign Language (TOEFL) is required for all applicants who are not U.S. citizens and for whom English is a second language. EXCEPTION: The TOEFL examination will be waived for students who have graduated with a baccalaureate or higher degree from a U.S. institution at time of application. Applicants must receive a minimum score of 550 (paper-based); 213 (computer-based); or 79 (internet-based). TOEFL must be taken within 3 years of applying.

*VMCAS Participation:* full

*Accepts International Students?* yes

## ADDITIONAL INFORMATION

*Additional requirements:* All applicants are required to complete the LMU-CVM Supplemental Application which will be available on the LMU-CVM website after the 2014-2015 VMCAS application cycle opens.

*Application Deadline:* 10/2/2014

# LOUISIANA STATE UNIVERSITY

Email Address: svmadmissions@lsu.edu
Website: http://www.vetmed.lsu.edu/admissions

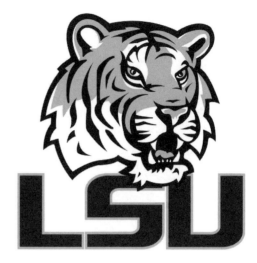

## SCHOOL DESCRIPTION

The Louisiana State University campus is located in Baton Rouge, which has a population of more than 500,000 and is a major industrial city, a thriving port, and the state's capital. Since it is located on the Mississippi River, Baton Rouge was a target for domination by Spanish, French, and English settlers. The city bears the influence of all three cultures and offers a range of choices in everything from food to architectural design. Geographically, Baton Rouge is the center of south Louisiana's main cultural and recreational attractions. Equally distant from New Orleans and the fabled Cajun bayou country, there is an abundance of cultural and outdoor recreational activities. South Louisiana has a balmy climate that encourages lush vegetation and comfortable temperatures year round.

> Geographically, Baton Rouge is the center of south Louisiana's main cultural and recreational attractions.

The campus encompasses more than 2,000 acres in the southern part of Baton Rouge and is bordered on the west by the Mississippi River. The Veterinary Medicine Building, occupied in 1978, houses the academic departments, the veterinary library, and the Veterinary Teaching Hospital and Clinics. The school is fully accredited by the American Veterinary Medical Association.

## APPLICATION INFORMATION

For specific application information (availability, deadlines, fees, and VMCAS participation), please refer to the LSU SVM admissions website at www.vetmed.lsu.edu/admissions.

*Residency implications:* The LSU SVM accepts 55-60 in-state residents and has approximately 9 seats reserved for AR contract students. The remaining 18-23 seats are offered to non-resident students.

## SUMMARY OF ADMISSION PROCEDURES

*Timetable*

*Suggested last date to take GRE:* October 1

*VMCAS application deadline:* Tuesday, October 2, 2014 1:00 PM Eastern Time

*Supplemental application deadline:* October 15 (Supplemental Application Link: www.vetmed.lsu.edu /admissions)

*Supplemental application fee ($75) deadline:* October 15

*GRE score submission deadline:* November 15

*Date interviews are held:* February/March*

*Date acceptances mailed:* mid-March

*School begins:* mid-August

*Interview invitations are extended to a select number of Louisiana, Arkansas, and out of state applicants as determined by the LSU SVM Admissions Committee.

*Deposit (to hold place in class):* $500.00 for nonresidents only.

*Deferments:* considered on a case-by-case basis.

## EVALUATION CRITERIA

The approximate components of the evaluation scoring are:
Objective evaluation:
GPA required courses: 29%
GPA last 45 hours: 18%
Test scores: 18%

## PREREQUISITES FOR ADMISSION

| Course Description | Number of Hours/Credits | Necessity |
| --- | --- | --- |
| General Biology | 8 | Required |
| Microbiology (w/lab) (1) | 4 | Required |
| Physics | 6 | Required |
| General Chemistry | 8 | Required |
| Organic chemistry | 3 | Required |
| Biochemistry (2) | 3 | Required |
| English Composition | 6 | Required |
| Speech Communication | 3 | Required |
| Mathematics | 5 | Required |
| Electives | 20 | Required |

*Subjective evaluation:*

Animal/veterinary experience, references: 15% (min. of 3 required, one by a veterinarian), essay, knowledge of profession, etc

Personal interview: 10%

Committee evaluation: 10%

## ENTRANCE REQUIREMENTS

*Required undergraduate GPA:* the minimum acceptable GPA for required coursework is 3.00 on a 4.00 scale. The mean GPA of the most recent entering class at the time of acceptance was 3.77.

*AP credit policy:* must appear on official college transcripts and be equivalent to the appropriate college-level coursework.

*Is a Bachelor's Degree Required?* no

*Is this an International School?* no

## ESTIMATED TUITION

*Estimated Tuition Resident:* $19,552

*Estimated Tuition Contract:* $19,552

*Estimated Tuition Non-Resident:* $45,352

## AVAILABLE SEATS

*Resident:* 60

*Contract:* 9

*Non-Resident:* 23

## TEST REQUIREMENTS

*Standardized examinations:* The GRE revised General Test is required. The scores must be received no later than November 15. Note: All applicants must take the GRE revised General Test.

*VMCAS Participation:* full

*Accepts International Students?* yes

## ADDITIONAL INFORMATION

*Application Deadline:* 10/2/2014

# MICHIGAN STATE UNIVERSITY

Email Address: admiss@cvm.msu.edu
Website: http://www.cvm.msu.edu

## SCHOOL DESCRIPTION

Michigan State University's campus is bordered by the city of East Lansing, which offers sidewalk cafes, restaurants, shops, and convenient mass transit. The campus is traversed by the Red Cedar River and has many miles of bike paths and walkways. This park-like setting provides an ideal venue in which MSU's 48,906 students may enjoy outdoor concerts and plays, canoeing, and cross-country skiing. The campus is located in East Lansing, three miles east of Michigan's capitol in Lansing. It sits on a 5,200-acre campus with 2,100 acres in existing or planned development. There are 532 buildings which include 103 academic buildings.

> Michigan State University is a national leader in state-of-the-art technology and facilities.

The college is a national leader in state-of-the-art technology and facilities. The Information Technology Center empowers and assists students, faculty, and staff with the knowledge needed to fulfill everyday computer tasks. The Veterinary Teaching Hospital has one of the largest caseloads in the country. Outstanding faculty are involved in teaching veterinary students, providing patient treatment and diagnostic services, and conducting veterinary research.

There are four state-of-the art facilities that have been added in the past few years to our medical complex. They are the new Diagnostic Center for Population and Animal Health (DCPAH), the Center for Comparative Oncology, the Mary Anne McPhail Equine Performance Center, and the Matilda R. Wilson Pegasus Critical Care Center and the Training Center for Dairy Professionals. For information about these centers, please visit the links provided below.

http://animalhealth.msu.edu/

http://cvm.msu.edu/hospital/services/comparative-oncology-center

http://cvm.msu.edu/hospital/special-facilities/Plone//research/research-centers/mcphail-equine-performance-center

http://cvm.msu.edu/departments/large-animal-clinical-sciences/services-research-centers/pegasus-critical-care-center?searchterm=pegasus

## APPLICATION INFORMATION

For specific application information (pre-requisite science courses, deadlines, fees, and VMCAS participation), please refer to our website: http://cvm.msu.edu

*Residency implications:* priority is given to Michigan residents. Up to 35 positions are filled with nonresident and international applicants.

## SUMMARY OF ADMISSION PROCEDURES

*VMCAS application deadline:* Thursday, October 2, 2014 1:00 PM Eastern Time

Electronic evaluations to VMCAS, Thursday, October 2, 2014 1:00 PM Eastern Time

GRE taken by September 30. The dateline to received GRE scores is December 15

All transcripts submitted of courses taken prior the October 2 deadline should be submitted to VMCAS by October 2

## PREREQUISITES FOR ADMISSION

| Course Description | Number of Hours/Credits | Necessity |
|---|---|---|
| English Composition | 3 | Required |
| Social and Behavioral Sciences | 6 | Required |
| Humanities | 6 | Required |
| General Inorganic Chemistry (with Laboratory) | 3 | Required |
| Organic Chemistry (with laboratory) | 6 | Required |
| Biochemistry (upper division) | 3 | Required |
| General Biology (with laboratory) | 6 | Required |
| College Algebra and Trigonometry | 3 | Required |
| College Physics (with laboratory) | 8 | Required |
| Nutrition | 3 | Required |
| Genetics | 3 | Required |
| Cell Biology (eukaryotic) | 3 | Required |
| Microbiology (with laboratory) | 4 | Required |

International transcripts must be evaluated by a translation service such us World Education Services (WES), Josef Silny or the American Association of Collegiate Registrars an Admission Officers, Foreign Education Credential Service (AACRAO). It is recommended that transcript(s) be submitted to the translation service at least one month prior to the deadline of October 2

*Deposit (to hold place in class):* (none refundable) $500.00 for residents; $1,000.00 for nonresidents.

Deferments are rare.

## ENTRANCE REQUIREMENTS

*Required undergraduate GPA:* No minimum required. The mean cumulative GPA for the entering class (2013) was 3.56 on a 4.00 scale.

*AP credit policy:* AP credit(s) must appear on an official transcript and be equivalent to appropriate college-level coursework.

*Is a Bachelor's Degree Required?* no

*Is this an International School?* no

## ESTIMATED TUITION

*Estimated Tuition Resident:* $27,048

*Estimated Tuition Contract:* $0

*Estimated Tuition Non-Resident:* $52,206

## AVAILABLE SEATS

*Resident:* 79

*Contract:* 0

*Non-Resident:* 34

## TEST REQUIREMENTS

*Standardized examinations:* The Graduate Record Examination (GRE), general test, is required to be taken no later than September 30. Test scores older than 5 years will not be accepted.

*VMCAS Participation:* full

*Accepts International Students?* yes

## ADDITIONAL REQUIREMENTS AND CONSIDERATIONS

Evaluation of written application (including veterinary/research experience)

Supplemental application: A link to the supplemental application will be sent to the applicant

Letters of recommendation (3 submitted by October 2, 2014 at 1:00 PM Eastern Time through VMCAS; 1 must be completed by a veterinarian)

Interview by the discretion of the Committee on Student Admissions)

## 2013-2014 ADMISSIONS SUMMARY

*Number of Applicants*

*Resident:* 236

*Nonresident/International:* 625

*Total:* 861

*Number of New Entrants*

*Resident:* 79

*Nonresident/International:* 34

*Total:* 113

## EXPENSES AND FEES

*Resident:* $27,048

*Nonresident:* $53,244

## EARLY ADMISSION PROGRAM

The Veterinary Scholars Admission Program has been established by the College of Veterinary Medicine in cooperation with the Honors College at Michigan State University. This program provides admission opportunity for students who wish to enter the four year professional veterinary medicine degree program after earning a bachelor's degree. The bachelor's degree program must include advanced and enriched coursework representing scholarly interest and achivements. Enrollment at MSU and membership in the Honors College are required to be eligible for this option. For information on Honors College membership, contact: Honors College, 105 Eustace-Hall, 468 E. Circle Drve, Michigan State University, East Lansing, MI 48824; telephone (517) 355-2326; or visit their website at http://honorscollege.msu.edu/.

## PRODUCTION MEDICINE PATHWAY

The Production Medicine Scholars Pathway has been established by the College of Veterinary Medicine in cooperation with the department of Animal Sciences at Michigan State University. This pathway is available to MSU Animal Science students who complete, in addition to the minimum pre-veterinary medicine requirements, a bachelor's degree in Animal Sciences with a concentration in production animal medicine. The concentration is designed to prepare students for a career in herd based, agricultural veterinary practice. The pathway provides an early admission option for Michigan State University students planing to earn a baccalaureate degree in Animal Science with a concentration in production medicine. Successful applicants must have a strong academic and non-academic credentials, a demonstrated interest in food animal production medicine and agricultural veterinary medicine. Additional information about the pathway may be obtained from 1250 Anthony Hall, 474 S. Shaw Lane, Department of Animal Science, Michigan State University, East Lansing, MI 48824 or visit the website: http://www.ans.msu.edu

## DUAL DEGREE PROGRAMS

Combined DVM-MPH degree program available

Combined online DVM/MS in Food Safety available

*Application Deadline:* 10/2/2014

### Why do you want to be a veterinarian?

I grew up on a small farm in Northern Michigan that specialized in pasture-raised meat and breeding Shire Draft horses. From a young age, my parents instilled in me a duty to my animals. They provide meat, recreation, and friendship to us as humans, and in return we have a responsibility to give them the best care possible. It is their purity of affection that led me to need to be a veterinarian. Knowing that my horse, for example, depended on me to help him heal from an injury or fever always made waiting for the vet torturous growing up—I wanted to help, but I couldn't be sure if what I did would make it better or worse. As a vet, I am hoping that even if I may not always have the answers, I will be much more able to ease their suffering.

### What did you do as an applicant to prepare for veterinary school?

I was very thorough and detailed in my experiences that I listed. I also made sure to go through the classes I took in undergrad and list some of my experiences from them in VMCAS (e.g., dissecting ascarids, fish, and oysters in biology; breeding fruit flies in genetics; etc.). Since coming to vet school, it has become obvious to me that not all courses at different universities cover the same material or offer the same experiences, so if you did something that you feel is unique in your class, be sure to list it, since details like that will not show up on your transcript.

### What advice would you give to applicants or those considering veterinary school?

Be thorough and honest about your experiences. Do use action words and represent yourself in a positive light. Have someone who has gone through the process recently look over your application to give you feedback. It's also really helpful to have someone supporting you who recently started vet school. The year you apply is extremely stressful, so it makes a difference having someone who has made it through the other side to give you perspective. Also, be sure to call the schools you are interested in to check your application status. I know a few people who didn't get into vet school their first attempt because their application was lost, so take steps to avoid that.

### What helped make the transition to veterinary school easier?

If finances allow, go to your visit day and move in to the area at least a week before classes start. If you end up being able to visit, make friends with one of the vet students there so you can contact him or her with any questions before moving in and during the transition. Breathe. The first couple of weeks can be stressful, but don't tear yourself down. Also, don't compare yourself to your classmates. This only adds unnecessary stress. Use them as a resource and share your knowledge with others. Everyone should work together to learn the material, not bring each other down. Do not become a vet because you want to make money. Become a vet because you can't imagine living any other way. It is very rewarding and remarkable work, and we are able to change the lives of so many, but it is demanding as well. As for personal relationships, keep in touch with family and friends. Especially if you live far from home, it may be difficult to find time to call them sometimes, but they will help to keep you grounded. Finally, make friends with upperclassmen, especially fourth years. By that time, they have the scoop on the whole school and how it works. Their advice is invaluable.

### What is your advice on financial aid?

Go to an in-state school. I didn't. I do not regret my decision, but if you choose to go out of state and turn down an in-state option, you must have a plan to get out of debt. Do not go in blindly. The job market right now is extremely competitive, and vets coming out of school make very little money. Debt forgiveness plans are wonderful *if* you meet the requirements and *if* the government can continue to afford them, but just remember that when that debt is forgiven you have to pay taxes on it. Work during school and during breaks. There are also many ways to find paid experiences during the summer. Your school will have several opportunities, as will your professors, as will the national species organizations that hopefully you join (e.g., AABP, AAEP, etc). Never waste a break. You need varied experiences to set you apart. Be creative in what you choose.

### What advice do you have for students who are considering applying to veterinary school?

Most of my classmates are on their second careers, and some already have master's or additional degrees. When I first found this out, I was pretty intimidated. After meeting them and making friends, however, I have come to appreciate their added life experience. It doesn't matter how long you have wanted to be a vet. If you have the passion to see it through, you will be successful.

# MIDWESTERN UNIVERSITY

Email Address: admissaz@midwestern.edu
Website: http://www.midwestern.edu/

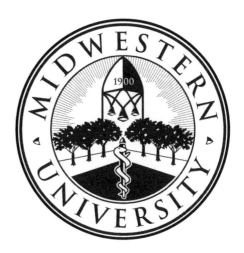

## SCHOOL DESCRIPTION

The Midwestern University College of Veterinary Medicine (MWU-CVM) presents to its students a four year program leading to the Doctor of Veterinary Medicine (DVM) degree. The first 8 quarters are a mix of classroom lectures, laboratories, simulation lab exercises with virtual clients and patients, and small group, student-centered learning experiences. Hands-on live animal contact begins in the first quarter and continues throughout the program. Quarters 9-13 involve diverse clinical training, both on campus (about 85%) and at external sites (about 15%). Three new buildings, including a 109,000 square foot small animal Veterinary Teaching Hospital and a roughly 36,000 square foot large animal/pathology facility, insure our students will begin their careers in state-ofthe-art surroundings.

> Three new buildings insure MWU-CVM students will begin their careers in state-of-the-art surroundings.

The MWU-CVM has received a Letter of Reasonable Assurance from the American Veterinary Medical Association (AVMA) Council on Education. This notification clears the way for the College to begin admitting students to its inaugural class of 100 students who are scheduled to matriculate in August 2014. It further indicates the University and College submitted a plan which successfully met the 11 standards required by the AVMA to become accredited. The program will be eligible for provisional accreditation in 2014 and full accreditation in 2018, upon graduation of the first class.

## APPLICATION INFORMATION

The CVM utilizes the Veterinary Medical College Application Service (VMCAS). The VMCAS application is available online at www.aavmc.org. The VMCAS application cycle opens in June of each year. The official VMCAS application deadline is generally in the first week of October. Midwestern University Office of Admissions may require a supplemental application form to be completed. Students who do not apply through VMCAS, or who have not met the VMCAS deadlines, must apply directly to the Midwestern University Office of Admissions. The direct application cycle will begin the first week of October, and the application will be available online at www.midwestern.edu. Requests for withdrawing an application must be submitted in writing. In accordance with the Association of American Veterinary Medical Colleges acceptance deadline policy, students are not required to accept or reject an offer of admission until April 15. Students may accept or reject earlier if so inclined. If a signed letter accepting admission and the required deposit are not received by April 15, the offer of admission may be withdrawn.

## SUMMARY OF ADMISSION PROCEDURES

Students seeking admission to the CVM must submit the following documented evidence:

1. Completion of prerequisite coursework or plans to complete the coursework prior to matriculation. (Confirmed by official transcripts)
   a. Minimum science AND minimum total cumulative GPA of 2.75 on a 4.00 scale.
   b. No grade lower than a C in any course will be accepted for credit. (Pass/fail and satisfactory/ unsatisfactory grading is not acceptable in prerequisite science courses).

| Course Description | Number of Hours/Credits | Necessity |
| --- | --- | --- |
| Biology | 8 | Required |
| General Chemistry with Lab | 8 | Required |
| Organic Chemistry with Lab | 8 | Required |
| Mathematics | 6 | Required |
| Physics with Lab | 4 | Required |
| English Composition | 6 | Required |
| Science Electives | 8 | Required |

2. Completion of a minimum of 240 hours (6 weeks) of veterinary, health sciences, animal or biomedical research experience. Students with additional hours of work experience will present a stronger case for admission.
3. Competitive scores on the GRE General Test.
4. Three letters of recommendation. (Students may submit up to 6 letters of recommendation.)
    a. At least one of the letters must be from a veterinarian.
    b. The other letters can be from other veterinarians, or from pre-veterinary or science professors, or from someone who can testify to the integrity and ethical standards of the applicant.
    c. Letters written by family members are not acceptable.
    d. Letters must be submitted by evaluators. Letters submitted by students are not accepted by the Office of Admissions.
5. Although not required, a Bachelor's degree will make a candidate more competitive.

## ENTRANCE REQUIREMENTS

1. Demonstrate an understanding of the veterinary medical profession
2. Demonstrate service orientation through com-munity service or extracurricular activities
3. Have a proper motivation for and commitment to the veterinary profession as demonstrated by previous salaried work, volunteer work, or other life experiences.
4. Possess the oral and written communication skills necessary to interact with patients, clients, and colleagues
5. Pass the Midwestern University criminal background check

6. Abide by Midwestern University's Drug-Free Workplace and Substance Abuse Policy.
7. Meet the Technical Standards for the College (see below).

*Is a Bachelor's Degree Required?* no

*Is this an International School?* no

## ESTIMATED TUITION

*Estimated Tuition Resident:* $52,400

*Estimated Tuition Contract:* $52,400

*Estimated Tuition Non-Resident:* $52,400

## AVAILABLE SEATS

Resident:      100

## TEST REQUIREMENTS

GRE

*VMCAS Participation:* full

*Accepts International Students?* yes

## ADDITIONAL INFORMATION

Science electives include biochemistry, cell biology, physiology, microbiology, genetics, animal nutrition, etc. Student applications may be strengthened by inclusion of a biochemistry course.

Minimum of 64 total semester hours/96 quarter hours

*Application Deadline:* 10/2/2014

# UNIVERSITY OF MINNESOTA

University of Minnesota
College of Veterinary Medicine
Email Address: dvminfo@umn.edu
Website: http://www.cvm.umn.edu/students/prospective
-dvm-students/index.htm

UNIVERSITY OF MINNESOTA

## College of Veterinary Medicine

## SCHOOL DESCRIPTION

The University of Minnesota College of Veterinary Medicine prepares future leaders in companion animal, food animal, and public health practice, as well as research and education. University of Minnesota students benefit from one of the largest teaching hospitals in the country, as well as world renowned faculty in zoonotic diseases, comparative medicine, and population systems. The College offers state-of-the-art facilities, including the Veterinary Medical Center, Leatherdale Equine Center, and the Raptor Center, which in 1988 became the world's first facility designed specifically for birds of prey. Off-site facilities include farms throughout Minnesota and around the world.

> Students gain hands-on experience throughout the entire program in clinical and professional skills courses.

The College of Veterinary Medicine is located on the 540-acre St. Paul campus. Students enjoy a small, intimate campus atmosphere of approximately 3,000 students while benefiting from the numerous amenities available within one of the nation's largest university systems.

The Twin Cities of Minneapolis and St. Paul have a combined population of approximately 2.5 million people and represents one of the largest metropolitan areas where a veterinary college is located. The Twin Cities is the cultural center for the region, abundant with outdoor recreational opportunities, and is repeatedly cited as one of the most livable metropolitan areas in the nation.

In 2013-14, the DVM program underwent a complete curriculum revision. During the first three years of the DVM program, students focus on the study of the normal animal, the pathogenesis of diseases and the prevention, alleviation and clinical therapy of diseases. Students gain hands-on experience throughout the entire program in clinical and professional skills courses.

The program concludes with thirteen months of clinical rotations in the Veterinary Medical Center, during which time students learn methods of veterinary care and develop skills needed for professional practice. Students can choose from over 80 rotation offerings. The fourth year includes up to twelve weeks of externship experiences at off-campus sites of the student's choice.

## APPLICATION INFORMATION

Application requirements include a complete VMCAS application, three electronic letters of reference submitted through VMCAS, official transcripts submitted through VMCAS, GRE examination scores, and an $85 application processing fee. The University of Minnesota College of Veterinary Medicine does not utilize a supplemental application.

The application, transcripts, and references are due to VMCAS by their respective deadlines.

All other application materials are due to the College by the application deadline of October 2, 2014, at 1 PM Eastern Time. For more application information, please visit http://www.cvm.umn.edu/education/prospective/home.html.

*Residency implications:* first priority is given to residents of Minnesota and residents of states with which a reciprocity or contract agreement exists (North Dakota and South Dakota). Residents of other states are

| PREREQUISITES FOR ADMISSION | | |
| --- | --- | --- |
| Course Description | Number of Hours/Credits | Necessity |
| English (2 courses) | 6 | Required |
| Algebra, Pre-Calculus, or Calculus | 3 | Required |
| General Chemistry w/ Labs (2 courses, plus 2 labs) | 6 | Required |
| Organic Chemistry w/ Lab | 3 | Required |
| Bichemistry | 3 | Required |
| General Biology w/ Lab | 3 | Required |
| Zoology w/ Lab | 3 | Required |
| Genetics | 3 | Required |
| Microbiology w/ Lab | 3 | Required |
| Physics w/ Lab (2 courses, plus 2 labs) | 6 | Required |
| Liberal Education: Arts and Humanities (2 courses) | 6 | Required |
| Liberal Education: Social Science and History (2 courses) | 6 | Required |

encouraged to apply. International applicants are only considered if their prerequisite coursework has been completed at a U.S. or Canadian college or university. The University of Minnesota will accept 102 students into the program each year. Approximately 55 of the 102 seats are reserved for resident/reciprocity eligible applicants. Approximately 47 seats are held for non-resident applicants.

## SUMMARY OF ADMISSION PROCEDURES

*Timetable*

*VMCAS application deadline:* Thursday, October 2, 2014 at 1:00 PM Eastern Time

*Date acceptances mailed:* mid-February

*School begins:* last week of August

*Deposit (to hold place in class):* $500.00

*Deferments:* can be requested for extenuating circumstances that warrant a 1-year delay in admission. Requests to defer submitted after July 15 will not be considered.

## EVALUATION CRITERIA

Objective measures of educational background

• GPA in prerequisite coursework

• GPA in most recent 45-semester credits

• GRE Test scores

Behavioral interviews

Subjective measures of personal experience

• Employment record

• Extracurricular and/or community service activities

• Leadership abilities

• References

• Maturity/reliability

• Animal/veterinary knowledge, experience, and interest

## 2013-2014 ADMISSIONS SUMMARY

*Number of Number of Applicants / New Entrants*

*Residents:* 179/47 admitted

*Non-Resident:* 782/55 admitted

*Total:* 961/102 admitted

The figures for new entrants include students taking delayed admission from the previous year.

*Includes residents of North and South Dakota

## EXPENSES FOR THE 2013-2014 ACADEMIC YEAR

*Tuition and fees*

*Residents:* $33,880*

*Nonresidents:* $58,346*

*This includes all tuition, fees, and one calendar year of health insurance costs (approximately $3,180). Health insurance is mandatory; students can petition out of insurance costs if proof of personal coverage is provided.

Students from Minnesota and South Dakota pay resident tuition rates. Students from North Dakota can apply to the state of North Dakota for tuition support. Approved North Dakota students pay resident tuition rates. North Dakota students not approved pay non-resident tuition rates. Students from all other states or international locations pay non-resident tuition rates.

Students may apply for residency after one year of enrollment.

## ENTRANCE REQUIREMENTS

All prerequisites must be graded at a C- or better. Math and science prerequisites courses must be recent within ten years of the application deadline.

*Liberal education requirements:* A minimum of four courses from the following areas of study: anthropology, art, economics, geography, history, humanities, literature (including foreign language literature), music, political science, psychology, public speaking, social science, sociology, theater.

*Required undergraduate GPA:* 2.75 minimum GPA required. The class of 2017 had a mean GPA of 3.65 (on a 4.00 scale) for required courses and 3.74 for the last 60 quarter-hour or 45 semester-hour credits of coursework prior to admission.

*AP credit policy:* must appear on official college transcripts and be equivalent to the appropriate college-level coursework.

*Course completion deadline:* prerequisite courses must be completed by the end of the spring term (not later than June 15) of the academic year in which application is made. No more than five prerequisite science courses may be pending completion during the fall and spring semesters of the application cycle. Science laboratory courses are not included in the count of five.

*Standardized examinations:* Graduate Record Examination (GRE), general test, is required. Results must be received by the College by the application deadline. The mean combined score for the verbal and quantitative sections of the GRE for the class of 2017 was 311. When scheduling your exam, confirm your test date will allow enough time for results to be delivered by the application deadline. Send test results to institution code 6904.

*Is a Bachelor's Degree Required?* no

*Is this an International School?* no

## ESTIMATED TUITION

*Estimated Tuition Resident:* $33,880

*Estimated Tuition Contract:* n/a

*Estimated Tuition Non-Resident:* $58,346

## AVAILABLE SEATS

*Resident:* 55

*Contract:* n/a

*Non-Resident:* 47

## TEST REQUIREMENTS

Graduate Record Exam

*VMCAS Participation:* full

*Accepts International Students?* yes

## ADDITIONAL INFORMATION

*Application Deadline:* 10/2/2014

# FOURTH-YEAR PROFILE: COURTNEY MARTIN

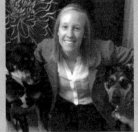

**What has been your favorite thing about attending veterinary school so far?**
My favorite thing has been at the end of each year realizing how much I have learned, how many amazing experiences I have been able to participate in, and how many wonderful people and animals I have had the chance to work with. Just today I was thinking about how fast time has gone by, how much has already been accomplished, and how truly fulfilling, however difficult, these last few years have been.

**What advice do you have for prospective veterinary school applicants?**
My advice would be to try to get as much veterinary exposure as possible prior to starting veterinary school. I worked in a mixed animal practice as an animal assistant the year before I started veterinary school and gained invaluable perspective. Once starting veterinary school, I felt like I had some type of context for the information being taught and an understanding for how this knowledge would be applicable to me in the near future. I think the best motivation to keep pushing through the long hours of studying in the first few years was to remember why all this information would be so important.

**What extracurricular activities have you been involved in during veterinary school?**
I was part of several clubs, including the equine, business, and shelter clubs. I also was the student representative for Bayer Animal Health during my second and third year, and have acted as a student ambassador for the University of Missouri veterinary program. I worked in a few research laboratories my first year and then in the ICU at our equine hospital as part of the after-hours student staff.

**What was the biggest challenge you faced during veterinary school?**
One of the biggest challenges I have faced during veterinary school has been finding a healthy balance. Although totally worth it, both the classroom and hands-on clinic time are mentally and physically exhausting, with many long days at school and then often many more hours spent at home studying or finishing clinical paperwork. I think maintaining a healthy social life and knowing when you need to take a break are important keys to a successful and enjoyable veterinary school experience.

**What advice do you have for other students who are currently in veterinary school?**
My advice would be to try to expose yourself to as many different opportunities as possible. While I have already accepted an equine position for next year, I do not know what the future will hold and what other job opportunities may arise. Also, you never know what things may interest or not interest you if you do not try a variety of things. Thus, when choosing externship opportunities, I have chosen a diverse array, including spay/neuter clinics, equine private practice, a veterinarian with mainly a cattle practice, and mixed animal practices.

**Why do you want to be a veterinarian?**
I love being outside, and I love caring for animals. As a child, I use to listen to James Herriot's stories on cassette tapes while falling asleep in bed. I was fascinated by the diversity of his day-to-day routine and knew I wanted to live out these stories. The first time I shadowed a large animal veterinary and he pulled out a silver bucket before we walked into the dairy barn, just like the ones from James Herriot used to describe in his stories, I knew this was the career for me.

**Are you taking advantage of any scholarship, loans, or loan repayment programs?**
In addition to taking out loans for veterinary school, I have been fortunate enough to receive several scholarships as well. I will not be taking advantage of a loan repayment program directly after graduating school, but I have thought about potentially applying to large animal loan forgiveness programs practicing in rural areas in the future.

# MISSISSIPPI STATE UNIVERSITY

Email Address: MSU-CVMAdmissions@cvm.msstate.edu
Website: http://www.cvm.msstate.edu

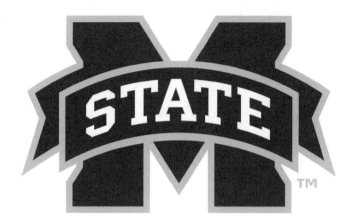

## SCHOOL DESCRIPTION

Starkville is home to more than 20,000 MSU students and their Bulldogs. Starkville is located in northeast central Mississippi and has a population of 24,000. Being a land-grant university, MSU is green and beautifully landscaped. The university includes 9 farms scattered throughout the state. The College of Veterinary Medicine (the Wise Center) was completed in 1982. The college includes 620 rooms on 8 acres, or 360,000 square feet, under one roof.

> The curriculum of the MSU-CVM is divided into 2 phases: Phase 1 or Pre-clinical and Phase 2 or Clinical.

The curriculum of the MSU-CVM is divided into 2 phases: Phase 1 or Pre-clinical (freshman and sophomore years) and Phase 2 or Clinical (junior and senior years).

Year 1 uses foundation courses to expose the student to important medical concepts and address multidisciplinary problems.

Year 2 is devoted to the study of clinical diseases and abnormalities of animal species. Surgery labs begin in the second year.

Year 3 is comprised of clinical rotations in the College's Animal Health Center, and elective courses.

Year 4 includes core rotations in internal medicine and ICU, large animal ambulatory, neurology, ophthalmology, and the Jackson Emergency/Referral Clinic.

The remainder of the fourth year is largely experiential and offers the student the opportunity to select among approved experiences in advanced clinical rotations, elective courses, or externships. The first 3 years of the curriculum are 9-10 months in length, while the fourth year is 12 months.

## APPLICATION INFORMATION

For specific application information (availability, deadlines, fees, and VMCAS participation), please refer to the contact information listed above.

*Residency implications:* Mississippi State accepts 40 Mississippi residents, 5 contract students from South Carolina, 7 contract students from West Virginia, and 33 non-resident applicants.

## SUMMARY OF ADMISSION PROCEDURES

*Timetable*

*VMCAS application deadline:* October 1, 2014, 1:00 PM Eastern Time

*GRE General Exam scores and supplemental application deadline:* October 1, 2014, 1:00 PM Eastern Time

*Date interviews are held:* January and February

*Date acceptances mailed:* February

*First-year classes begin:* early July

*Deposit (to hold place in class):* $500.00.

*Deferments:* requests are considered on an individual basis.

## EVALUATION CRITERIA

Grades (minimum competitive GPAs are typically 3.3-3.4)

Quality of academic program

| Prerequisites for Admission | | |
|---|---|---|
| Course Description | Number of Hours/Credits | Necessity |
| English Composition | 6 | Required |
| Speech or Technical Writing | 3 | Required |
| Mathematics (College Algebra or higher) | 6 | Required |
| General Biology and laboratory | 8 | Required |
| Microbiology with laboratory | 4 | Required |
| General Chemistry and laboratory | 8 | Required |
| Organic Chemistry and laboratory | 8 | Required |
| Biochemistry | 3 | Required |
| Physics (may be Trig-based) | 6 | Required |
| Advanced (upper-level) science electives | 12 | Required |
| Humanities, fine arts, social sciences and behavioral electives | 15 | Required |

## TEST SCORES

Animal/veterinary experience

Participation in extra-curricular and community service activities and outside employment

Leadership and interpersonal skills

References (3 required; one must be from a veterinarian)

Personal statement

Interview of applicants selected on basis of academic and non-academic criteria.

## ENTRANCE REQUIREMENTS

*Required undergraduate GPA:* a minimum overall GPA of 2.8 on a 4.0 scale. The minimum GPA must be maintained throughout the application process. The class of 2017 has an average undergraduate GPA of 3.62.

At the time of application, no grade lower than a C- is acceptable in any required course. Remediated and repeated courses must be completed before the application is submitted.

*AP credit policy:* must appear on official college transcripts and be equivalent to the appropriate college-level coursework.

*Is a Bachelor's Degree Required?* no

*Is this an International School?* no

## ESTIMATED TUITION

*Estimated Tuition Resident:* $18,782

*Estimated Tuition Contract:* $18,782

*Estimated Tuition Non-Resident:* $43,982

**Available Seats**

*Resident:* 40

*Contract:* 12

*Non-Resident:* 33

## TEST REQUIREMENTS

*Standardized examinations:* Graduate Record Exam (GRE), general test, is required (no minimum score) and is due at the school by October 1.

GRE must have been taken within 3 years of application deadline.

Students should schedule the GRE exam 30 days prior to deadline.

*VMCAS Participation:* full

*Accepts International Students?* yes

## ADDITIONAL INFORMATION

*DVM-PhD Program*
The mission of the MSU-CVM DVM-PhD program is to prepare exceptional students for careers as veterinary scientists to meet the nation's critical needs in ani-

mal and human health research. It is the intent of the MSU-CVM DVM-PhD program to provide the full rigor of training from the DVM and PhD degrees as if they were pursued separately. The program is designed to integrate the research and clinical training programs so that students will experience a logical progression and level of responsibility throughout the program. It is also the intent of the program to provide a system of moral and financial support for the students who have committed to it.

## APPLICATION PROCESS

The simultaneous pursuit of DVM and PhD degrees requires a highly motivated student who can handle a rigorous course load. Students seeking admission to this program go through a two-step interview process. The student is interviewed for admission into the DVM professional education program and the graduate program of the college. A student admitted to the DVM-PhD program takes graduate coursework and after two years begins the DVM professional education curriculum. Completion of the DVM-PhD program will require 7 years in most cases; however, this is 1 to 2 years shorter than the time required to complete both degrees if they were pursued separately.

## PROGRAM STRUCTURE

An applicant granted admission to the DVM-PhD program will initiate his/her PhD coursework in the upcoming summer or fall semester and will remain engaged in graduate work until the fall semester two years later. Students admitted to the DVM-PhD program will have a position reserved in the DVM program two years subsequent to starting the DVM-PhD program as long as the student progressed appropriately during the initial two years of the PhD program. Upon successful completion of graduate coursework (maintaining a 3.0 GPA), a successful preliminary defense, and acceptance of a research proposal in the format of a federal agency grant proposal by the student's PhD committee, the student will continue in the DVM-PhD program and begin the DVM professional curriculum. Once the student has entered the DVM curriculum, he or she will matriculate through the DVM program with the same class he/she enters the curriculum with. The final year of the program will be spent completing the PhD research, writing, and defending the dissertation.

## FINANCIAL SUPPORT

During semesters when a student is engaged in graduate coursework and/or dissertation research hours, he or she will receive a graduate stipend at the standard rate for MSU-CVM. The graduate stipend includes tuition waiver.

DVM-PhD students in good standing will receive a $40,000 tuition remission to be applied toward their DVM tuition.

## MSU-CVM EARLY ENTRY PROGRAM

The Early Entry Program is a unique program of the College of Veterinary Medicine (CVM) that allows high-achieving high school seniors to earn pre-acceptance (early, pre-approved acceptance) into the CVM.

Students who have an interest in veterinary medicine and meet application requirements during high school may apply for the Early Entry Program. If a student is accepted into this program, he/she begins undergraduate work at MSU after high school graduation, and completes the first three to four years of prerequisite courses, while also working toward completion of a bachelor's degree. After the student has completed all course requirements for the College of Veterinary Medicine, has remained in good standing, and has taken the GRE General Exam, he/she matriculates into the CVM as a pre-accepted student. The student does not make further application to the CVM.

Students applying for this program must have the following qualifications:
1. ACT composite score of 27 (SAT score of 1820 on new SAT); and
2. High school grade average of 90 (3.6 on a 4.0 scale)

In addition, the Early Entry Program Admissions Committee considers animal and veterinary experience, work experience, leadership qualities, and nontechnical skills and aptitudes (character, community service, etc.) as described in the applicant's written application to the Early Entry Program, and in the applicant's Letters of Recommendation (provided in the application).

Twenty-five positions are available each year. We normally receive 50 to 75 applications. Both Mississippi and out-of-state students are eligible for the program.

Applications for the Early Entry Program are available by October 1 each year, and are due for return by January 5. Applicants are notified of acceptance status by early February.

Applications are available online from October 1 through December 31. Please see the following website for the application and important information: http://www.cvm.msstate.edu/academics/early_entry_program.html

*Application Deadline:* 10/2/2014

# FIRST-YEAR PROFILE: DYLAN MICHAEL DJANI

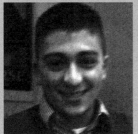

### Why do you want to be a veterinarian?
I am very interested in science and evolution, and veterinary medicine is a career where I am able to learn and apply science that will potentially benefit both humans and animals.

### What are your short-term and long-term goals?
For the short term, I am interested in pursuing summer research programs available at veterinary schools across the U.S. and building on existing relationships with mentors at my own school. My short-term goals should help me reach my long-term goal of becoming a veterinary specialist in some aspect of small animal medicine or surgery.

### What did you do as an applicant to prepare for veterinary school?
During my undergraduate years, I made sure to take advanced coursework that would directly benefit me during the preclinical phase of veterinary school, such as immunology and hematology, while also participating in two research projects. Regarding clinical experience, I worked primarily with a small animal veterinarian who watched me grow up and helped me branch out to the local emergency clinic and large animal veterinarian, allowing me to obtain a well-rounded basis for my veterinary school application.

### What advice would you give to applicants or those considering veterinary school?
Learn as much as you can about the various opportunities available to veterinary graduates, as there are a multitude of career paths that veterinarians can take, aside from traditional private practice. Preparing for veterinary school will give you a taste of the dedication required throughout the program, so making sure that veterinary medicine is the right fit is important.

### What helped make the transition to veterinary school easier?
The upperclassmen and faculty in veterinary school were phenomenal in making the transition easier. Everybody is willing to offer help and advice on a consistent basis.

### What is your advice on financial aid?
Student loans are in most cases inevitable, since veterinary school is of the professional caliber. I advise taking enough money to live on throughout the program in accordance with a budget. The program is demanding enough, and the last thing that any professional student wants to worry about is money. However, there are scholarships available to veterinary students to help mitigate costs, as well as loan repayment plans available for after graduation.

### What are you most excited about learning in veterinary school?
Now that I've been exposed to proper anatomy, I am looking forward to learning about surgical approaches to restore the proper anatomy during various diseases.

### What advice do you have for students who are considering applying to veterinary school?
Veterinary school was always a thought in the back of my mind growing up, but I was not certain until college that I wanted to attend. I think a thorough understanding of how professional school works influenced my decision, and that understanding did not come until my undergraduate years.

# UNIVERSITY OF MISSOURI

Email Address: seayk@missouri.edu
Website: https://cvmsecure.missouri.edu/admission

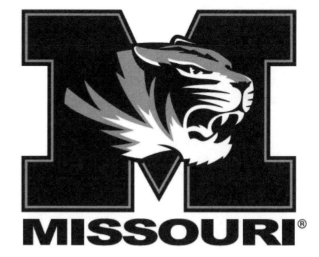

## SCHOOL DESCRIPTION

The University of Missouri is located among rolling forested hills north of the famous Lake of the Ozarks. Columbia is noted for its high quality of life and low cost of living and is consistently rated among the best cities to live in by Money Magazine. The city abounds with walking trails, 3,000 acres of state park lands, federal forests, and wildlife refuges. Columbia is located between Kansas City and St. Louis-cities that have major-league sports teams and other big-city recreational amenities. Columbia itself offers Big 12 Conference football, basketball, baseball and other sports. It boasts a 65,000-seat stadium, several 18-hole golf courses, and other indoor and outdoor recreation facilities. Our location near a metropolitan area provides a strong primary and referral small animal case load. Columbia's proximity to rural central Missouri results in an exceptional food animal and equine case load.

> The unique curriculum gives students 2 years of undiluted clinical experience before graduation.

MU, a major research university with 34,000 students, consists of 19 schools and colleges located on a 1,335-acre campus. The College of Veterinary Medicine is noted for its unique curriculum that gives students 2 years of undiluted clinical experience before graduation as opposed to the traditional 1-1.5 years. Students benefit from exposure to specialty medical areas such as clinical cardiology, neurology, orthopedics, ophthalmology, and oncology. Students also gain experience with advanced equipment such as a linear accelerator for treatment of cancer, MRI, state-of-the-art ultrasonography, extensive endoscopy equipment, cold lasers, a surgery room C-arm for radiography during surgical procedures, and others. MU is unique in having a medical school, nursing school, school of health-related professions, state cancer research center, the life sciences center, the second largest research animal diagnostic laboratory in the world and department of animal science on the same campus, thus enhancing teaching, research, and clinical services.

## APPLICATION INFORMATION

All applicants must apply through VMCAS and submit our Supplemental Application. For specific application information (availability, deadlines, fees, and VMCAS participation), please refer to the contact information listed above.

*Residency implications:* sixty seats are given to Missouri and sixty to non-residents. A total of 120 seats awarded each year. U.S. citizenship or permanent residency is required.

## SUMMARY OF ADMISSION PROCEDURES

*Early June, 2014:* VMCAS Application Opens

*September 2, 2014:* Transcripts due to VMCAS

*VMCAS application and all letters of reference due:* October 2, 2014 1:00 PM Eastern Time

*Supplemental Missouri application due:* October 3, 2014.

*January:* Out of state interviews held Feb-March: Missouri resident interviews held Date acceptances mailed: mid-April Orientation week: mid-August

*School begins:* late August

## PREREQUISITES FOR ADMISSION

| Course Description | Number of Hours/Credits | Necessity |
|---|---|---|
| English or Communication | 6 | Required |
| College algebra or higher | 3 | Required |
| Physics (complete sequence) | 5 | Required |
| Biological Science - not AS courses | 10 | Required |
| Humanities/Social Sciences | 10 | Required |
| Biochemistry with organic pre-req | 3 | Required |
| Electives | 10 | Required |

## ENTRANCE REQUIREMENTS

*Required undergraduate GPA:* Applicants must have a cumulative GPA of 3.00 or more on a 4.00 scale. The most recent entering class had a mean GPA of 3.77 at the time of acceptance.

*AP credit policy:* must appear on official college transcript and be equivalent to the appropriate college-level coursework.

*Is a Bachelor's Degree Required?* no

*Is this an International School?* no

## ESTIMATED TUITION

*Estimated Tuition Resident:* $22,522

*Estimated Tuition Contract:* pending

*Estimated Tuition Non-Resident:* $52,200

## AVAILABLE SEATS

*Resident:* 60

*Contract:* pending

*Non-Resident:* 60

## TEST REQUIREMENTS

*Standardized examinations:* The Medical College Admission Test (MCAT) or the Graduate Record Examination (GRE) general test is required. Test scores older than 3 years will not be accepted.

*VMCAS Participation:* full

*Accepts International Students?* no

## ADDITIONAL INFORMATION

Allows non-residents to gain residency after completing first year.

*Application Deadline:* 10/2/2014

# NORTH CAROLINA STATE UNIVERSITY

Email Address: cvm_dvm@ncsu.edu
Website: http://www.cvm.ncsu.edu

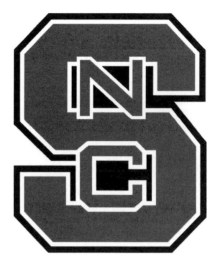

## SCHOOL DESCRIPTION

The North Carolina State University College of Veterinary Medicine is located on a 182-acre site in Raleigh, the state capital, which has a population of more than 400,000. The sandy shores of North Carolina's beautiful coastline are a short ride to the east, and the Great Smoky Mountains are to the west. The climate includes mild winters and warm summers.

The College of Veterinary Medicine opened in the fall of 1981 and encompasses 20 buildings on the main Centennial Biomedical Campus, including a teaching hospital, classrooms, animal wards, research and teaching laboratories, and an audiovisual area. The college has 140 faculty members and a capacity for 400 veterinary medical students with training for interns, residents, and graduate students.

> The College of Veterinary Medicine has 140 faculty members and a capacity for 400 veterinary medical students.

Construction started fall 2002 on the Centennial Biomedical Campus, which will be anchored by the College of Veterinary Medicine. An extension of the original NCSU Centennial Campus concept, the Centennial Biomedical Campus will house approximately 30 building sites. It will include an additional 1.6 million square feet of space over the next 25 years, resulting in a five-fold expansion of the current college and veterinary health complex. The two-year construction of the Randall B. Terry, Jr. Companion Animal Veterinary Medical Center was completed in June 2011. The Terry Center is considered the national model for excellence in companion animal medicine. The Terry Center offers cutting-edge technologies for imaging, cardiac care, cancer treatments, internal medicine, and surgery; has more than double the size of the former companion animal hospital; and accommodates the more than 22,000 cases referred to the CVM each year.

The Centennial Biomedical Campus will emphasize partnerships that work to bring academia, government and industry together. The focus of this campus is on biomedical applications, both to animals and humans. It will provide opportunities for industry and government researchers, entrepreneurs, clinical trial companies, as well as collaborations with other universities to work side by side with faculty and students at the College of Veterinary Medicine.

## APPLICATION INFORMATION

For specific application information (availability, deadlines, fees, and VMCAS participation), please refer to the contact information listed above.

*Residency implications:* priority is given to North Carolina residents. NOTE: The college increased its incoming class size from 80 to 100 starting with the 2012 admissions cycle. The current slot allocation is 80 resident and 20 nonresident slots. Non-resident admits are permitted to apply for residency for tuition purposes after the first 12 months in the program. NC State does accept international applicants.

## SUMMARY OF ADMISSION PROCEDURES

*VMCAS application deadline:* Tuesday, October 2, 2014 1:00 PM Eastern Time (VMCAS and NC State supplemental)

*Date acceptances mailed:* no later than April 1

*School begins:* August

## PREREQUISITES FOR ADMISSION

| Course Description | Number of Hours/Credits | Necessity |
|---|---|---|
| Animal Nutrition | 3 | Required |
| Biochemistry | 3 | Required |
| Biology | 4 | Required |
| Calculus or Logic | 3 | Required |
| Chemistry, General | 8 | Required |
| Chemistry, Organic | 8 | Required |
| Composition, Public Speaking or Communications | 6 | Required |
| Humanities and Social Sciences | 6 | Required |
| Microbiology | 4 | Required |
| Physics | 8 | Required |
| Statistics | 3 | Required |
| Genetics | 4 | Required |

*Deposit (to hold place in class):* $250.00.

*Deferments:* are considered for 1 year only, subject to Admissions Committee approval.

## EVALUATION CRITERIA

Selection for admission is a 2-phase process:

*Phase 1-Objective criteria:*

Required course GPA: 3.3 Resident, 3.4 Nonresident

Cumulative GPA: 3.0 Resident, 3.4 Nonresident

Last 45 credit hour GPA: 3.3 Resident, 3.4 Nonresident

GRE test score

Supplemental Application

*Phase 2-Subjective score:*

Applicant folder review by admissions committee

## ENTRANCE REQUIREMENTS

*AP credit policy:* must appear on official college transcripts with course name and credit hours and be equivalent to the appropriate college-level coursework.

*Is a Bachelor's Degree Required?* no

*Is this an International School?* yes

## ESTIMATED TUITION

*Estimated Tuition Resident:* $16,546

*Estimated Tuition Contract:* $0

*Estimated Tuition Non-Resident:* $39,599

## AVAILABLE SEATS

*Resident:* 80

*Contract:* 0

*Non-Resident:* 20

## TEST REQUIREMENTS

*Standardized examinations:* Graduate Record Examination (GRE), general test, is required. The scores must be received by the October 2 application deadline. There is no deadline to take the GRE.

*VMCAS Participation:* full

*Accepts International Students?* yes

## ADDITIONAL INFORMATION

*Application Deadline:* 10/2/2014

# THE OHIO STATE UNIVERSITY

Email Address: prospective@cvm.osu.edu
Website: vet.osu.edu/admissions

# THE OHIO STATE UNIVERSITY

## COLLEGE OF VETERINARY MEDICINE

## SCHOOL DESCRIPTION

The Ohio State University is located in Columbus, the state's capital and the nation's 15th largest city. Columbus has been rated the 7th best city in the nation for cost of living (Forbes Magazine) and one of the country's top-10 places to live (Money). Columbus offers all the cultural perks you would expect from a major metropolitan area including the #1 zoo in the country, according to the USA Travel Guide.

> The college is part of one of the largest and most comprehensive health sciences centers in the country.

The Ohio State University was founded in 1870 and is one of the nation's leading academic centers, consistently ranks as Ohio's best, and one of the nation's top-20 public universities. The campus consists of thousands of acres, hundreds of buildings, more than 15,000 faculty and staff, and more than 56,000 students.

The Veterinary Medical Center includes a Hospital for Companion Animals, Food Animal, and the Galbreath Equine Center. The patient load is one of the highest in the country and farmlands can be accessed 10 miles from campus. The Veterinary Medicine Academic Building has nearly 10,000 square feet of space and includes research labs, classrooms, a library, computer lab, and academic offices.

The Ohio State College of Veterinary Medicine is part of one of the largest and most comprehensive health sciences centers in the country that includes dentistry, medicine, nursing, optometry, pharmacy, public health, and veterinary medicine.

## APPLICATION INFORMATION

For specific application information (availability, deadlines, fees, and VMCAS participation), please refer to the contact information listed above.

*Residency implications:* applicants from all states will be considered. In-state and out-of state applicants are given equal consideration. We accept the top 162 students. We do accept international applicants.

## SUMMARY OF ADMISSION PROCEDURES

*VMCAS application deadline:* Thursday, October 2, 2014 1:00 PM Eastern Time

*Date interviews are held:* November-January

*Date acceptances mailed:* December-March

*School begins:* late August

*Deposit (to hold place in class):* $25.00 for residents; $300.00 (non-refundable fee) for contract and nonresident applicants.

*Deferments:* not considered

## EVALUATION CRITERIA

Academic Background (Cumulative GPA, GRE or MCAT scores, Last 45 credit hours, Pre-requisite science GPA and academic rigor)

File Review (Three references, Veterinary and Animal Experience - diversity & depth, personal statement)

Interview

Eligible applicants are interviewed and evaluated by members of the Admissions Committee.

**PREREQUISITES FOR ADMISSION**

| Course Description | Semester Units | Necessity |
|---|---|---|
| English | 3 | Required |
| General chemistry (with lab) | 10 | Required |
| Organic chemistry | 8 | Required |
| Biochemistry | 5 | Required |
| Biology | 8 | Required |
| Genetics | 3 | Required |
| Microbiology (with lab) | 4 | Required |
| Mathematics (algebra and trigonometry) | 5 | Required |
| General physics (with lab) | 10 | Required |
| Humanities and social sciences | 14 | Required |
| Electives | 8 | Required |
| Physiology | 3 | Recommended |
| Public speaking/communication | 3 | Recommended |

**Number of hours provided as a guideline. In assessing course content for equivalency, actual hours may vary for your institution. In some cases a multiple course series may be needed to fulfill prerequisite coursework.

**At some institutions, the prerequisite for biochemistry is two semesters/quarters. When Biochemistry is offered as a series, both courses in the series must be completed.

## Humanities and Social Sciences

Recommended Coursework:

Writing/speech – courses that emphasize written and/or verbal communication

Social Sciences – courses such as history, economics, anthropology, psychology, etc.

Humanities – courses in art, music, drama, literature, languages, etc.

Diversity/Ethics – courses that focus on the culture, history and/or current circumstances of different populations.

Electives: Elective courses are at the student's discretion, after consultation with an advisor. Recommended electives include embryology, immunology, anatomy, physiology, histology, animal science courses including nutrition.

Advanced Placement - In order to receive credit for AP courses, they must be listed on official transcripts from a college or university you have attended.

## ENTRANCE REQUIREMENTS

*Required undergraduate GPA:* the minimum GPA to be considered is 3.0 on a 4.0 scale. The most recent entering class had a mean overall GPA of 3.68 and a science GPA of 3.54. Prerequisite GPA is evaluated as well as last 45 semester or quarter hours.

*AP credit policy:* AP credit given if course is listed on official transcript.

*Is a Bachelor's Degree Required?* no

*Is this an International School?* no

## COURSE COMPLETION DEADLINE

Admission to the OSU College of Veterinary Medicine requires completion of the required prerequisites listed above or their equivalents from any accredited college or university. No more than one required prerequisite course may remain to be completed by the end of autumn semester of the academic year in which you apply; that course must be completed by the end of spring semester of the academic year in which you apply.

## ESTIMATED TUITION

*Estimated Tuition Resident:* $29,163

*Estimated Tuition Contract:* $0

*Estimated Tuition Non-Resident:* $63,291

Tuition is subject to change.

*For tuition purposes, nonresident students can apply for residency after completing their first year at the Ohio State University.

## AVAILABLE SEATS

*Resident:* Up to 100

*Contract:* 0

*Non-Resident:* up to 80

## TEST REQUIREMENTS

*Standardized examinations:* Graduate Record Examination (GRE) general test or the Medical College Admission (MCAT) test is required. Most applicants choose to take the GRE. Tests must be taken by September 30. Test scores must be received no later than October 1 of the year of application. GRE Code: 1592.

*VMCAS Participation:* full

*Accepts International Students?* yes

## ADDITIONAL INFORMATION

*Application Deadline:* 10/2/2014

# PRE-VETERINARIAN PROFILE: BRITTANY SENECAL

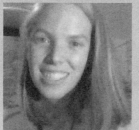

**YEAR OF GRADUATION**
2014

**Why are you interested in applying to veterinary school?**
I grew up in the family pet stores and have worked with reptiles, fish, small mammals, birds, dogs, and cats. Their health has always been the number one concern for us, so I learned from a young age what helps and hinders an animal's health. Becoming a vet just seemed to be the only choice I wanted to pursue from a very young age, and that desire has only increased the older I have become and the more involved in the stores I have become.

**What type of veterinary medicine are you interested in pursuing?**
When I entered my undergrad, I wanted to work on horses. Now, as a senior, I'm stuck between canine genetics and emergency medicine. Honestly, I am not sure what I want to do and just want to try a bunch of different things before I make up my mind.

**What did you major in during undergrad?**
I majored in general biology.

**What are your short-term and long-term goals?**
Short-term is graduation, possible acceptance into schools this application cycle (already have one interview!), and continuing my education. Even if I am not accepted this cycle, I will continue taking classes for another year as well as work for a local vet and volunteer at a local no-kill shelter. Long-term is make it through vet school, decide what I want to do with that education, and go from there.

**What are you doing as an applicant/pre-vet to prepare for veterinary school?**
My preparation started back in high school. I took 11 AP classes and came in with 28 credits to my undergrad institution. Because I didn't have to take any history or English classes, I was able to take classes that I would not have had time for, such as Parasitology, Mammalogy, and Animal Breeding and Reproduction. I also only had three semesters under 16 credit hours. I saw my adviser at least once a week, was active in various clubs, and also worked so I didn't have any loans from my undergrad.

**What extracurricular activities are you involved in currently?**
I have been in the school's pre-vet club all four years, serving as vice president and president junior and senior year. Last year I became active in the residence life association and became an RA.

**Have you shadowed or worked with any veterinarians in preparation to apply to vet school?**
I did shadow a veterinarian for a summer who my mom knew through our pet stores. It was a small animal clinic that mostly tended to dogs and cats, but one of the vets worked with reptiles, birds, and small mammals. I shadowed mainly one vet, but if there was an interesting or unique case one of the other doctors was working with, they would let me tag along for those. I helped with everything from cleaning to observing fecals to observing surgeries.

**What characteristics are you looking for in a veterinary school?**
My main goal is my in-state school simply on the basis of money. A part of being a veterinarian is acknowledging that you have a massive amount of debt that will need to be paid back. My in-state school is $10,000 less a year than my second pick, and every penny counts. After cost, my main concern was program orientation, since I do not have a path picked out. I chose schools that had a lot of variety in programs from small animal, to research, to exotics, and more.

**What advice do you have for students who are considering applying to veterinary school?**
Look at school information now! If you are going to stick to your guns and go for it, it is never too early to look at school information. Secondly, pick the major you want to do. There is no pre-vet major. If I could do it again, I would be a fine arts major with a minor in biology. I enjoyed my science classes fine, but I enjoy art more. Third, when picking your undergrad institution, look at what opportunities the school offers you. Does it have an active pre-vet club that can help you get animal, veterinary, or research hours? Does the school help you find internships? Grades are not everything in vet school, and if an undergrad institution does not help you find opportunities, then consider somewhere else.

# OKLAHOMA STATE UNIVERSITY

Email Address: dvm@okstate.edu
Website: http://www.cvhs.okstate.edu

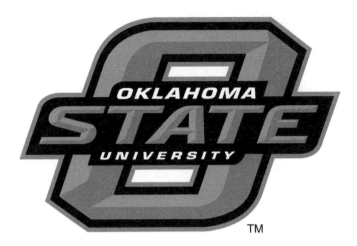

## SCHOOL DESCRIPTION

Oklahoma State University is located in Stillwater, which has a population of about 46,000. Stillwater is in north central Oklahoma about 65 miles from Oklahoma City and 69 miles from Tulsa. The campus is exceptionally beautiful, with modified Georgian-style architecture in the new buildings. It encompasses 840 acres and more than 60 major academic buildings.

Three major buildings form the veterinary medicine complex. The oldest, McElroy Hall, houses the William E. Brock Memorial Library and Learning Center, as well as classrooms and laboratories. The Boren Veterinary Medical Teaching Hospital provides modern facilities for both academic and clinical instruction. Completing the triad is the Oklahoma Animal Disease Diagnostic Laboratory, which provides teaching resources for students in the professional curriculum and diagnostic services to Oklahoma agriculture and industry. The College of Veterinary Medicine is fully accredited by the American Veterinary Medical Association. Faculty members in the three academic departments share responsibility for the curriculum. These departments are Veterinary Clinical Sciences, Veterinary Pathobiology, and Physiological Sciences.

> Faculty members in the three OSU academic departments share responsibility for the curriculum.

## APPLICATION INFORMATION

For specific application information (availability, deadlines, fees, and VMCAS participation), please refer to the contact information listed above.

*Residency implications:* entering class size is 82, which includes 58 Oklahoma residents and 24 non-residents. Some non-resident contract seats are available through AR and DE. International applications are accepted.

## SUMMARY OF ADMISSION PROCEDURES

*Timetable*

*VMCAS application deadline:* Thursday, October 2, 2014 1:00 PM Eastern Time

*Date interviews held:* February

*Date acceptances mailed:* March

*School begins:* mid-August

*Deposit (to hold place in class):* resident, $100.00; nonresident, $500.00

## EVALUATION CRITERIA

The admission procedure consists of evaluation of both academic and nonacademic criteria. The Admissions Committee considers all factors in the applicant's file, but the following are especially important: academic achievement; familiarity with the profession and sincerity of interest; recommendations; test scores; extracurricular activities; character, personality, and general fitness and commitment for a career in veterinary medicine. The committee selects those applicants considered most capable of excelling as veterinary medical students and who possess the greatest potential for success in the veterinary medical profession.

## PREREQUISITES FOR ADMISSION

| Course Description | Number of Hours/Credits | Necessity |
|---|---|---|
| Biochemistry | 3 | Required |
| Biology/Zoology | 8 | Required |
| English Composition 1 & 2 | 6 | Required |
| English Elective | 3 | Required |
| Genetics | 3 | Required |
| Humanities/Social Science | 6 | Required |
| Inorganic Chemistry | 8 | Required |
| Math (College Algebra - No Statistics) | 3 | Required |
| Organic Chemistry | 8 | Required |
| Physics 1 & 2 | 8 | Required |
| Microbiology | 4 | Required |
| Animal Nutrition | 3 | Required |

## ENTRANCE REQUIREMENTS

*Required undergraduate GPA:* a minimum GPA of 2.8 (on a 4.00 scale) is required in prerequisite courses. The mean cumulative GPA of the 2013 entering class was 3.484.

*AP credit policy:* AP credit accepted if documented on college transcript.

*Is a Bachelor's Degree Required?* no

*Is this an International School?* no

## ESTIMATED TUITION

*Estimated Tuition Resident:* $18,340 (tuition + fees for one full year)

*Estimated Tuition Contract:* $0

*Estimated Tuition Non-Resident:* $39,620 (tuition + fees for one full year)

## AVAILABLE SEATS

*Resident:* 58

*Contract:* 0

*Non-Resident:* 24

## TEST REQUIREMENTS

*Standardized examinations:* Graduate Record Examination (GRE), general test is required. The class of 2017 had mean scores of 153 verbal, 151 quantitative, and analytical of 4.0. Scores must be received by November 15, 2014 to the OSU-CVHS Student Services Office.

*VMCAS Participation:* full

*Accepts International Students?* yes

## ADDITIONAL INFORMATION

*Application Deadline:* 10/2/2014

# OREGON STATE UNIVERSITY

Email Address: cvmadmissions@oregonstate.edu
Website: http://vetmed.oregonstate.edu/

OSU
**Oregon State**
UNIVERSITY

## SCHOOL DESCRIPTION

The Oregon State University College of Veterinary Medicine is the smallest DVM program in the U.S. admitting only 56 students per year. Hands-on education is an important aspect to how our students learn and develop their knowledge of the profession. Our partnership with the Oregon Humane Society provides an opportunity for students to continue growing their skill level and confidence in their ability to perform as professionals. Students at OSU work in state-of-the-art facilities alongside our world-class faculty, including specialists in cardiology, oncology, imaging, and rehabilitation. The individual attention our students get from faculty and hospital staff is, in part, why year after year 100% percent of our students pass their board exams.

> Hands-on education is an important aspect to how our students learn and develop knowledge of the profession.

## APPLICATION INFORMATION

All components of the Oregon State DVM application are due by October 2. No materials will be accepted after this date including transcripts and GRE scores.

## SUMMARY OF ADMISSION PROCEDURES

Steps to apply for admission to Oregon State University College of Veterinary Medicine:
1. Begin the VMCAS application process

2. Request all transcripts be sent direct to VMCAS, they must be received by September 2, 2014.
   VMCAS Transcripts
   P O Box 9126
   Watertown, MA 02471
3. Submit GRE scores via ETS to Oregon State University College of Vet Med code: 4565 (scores must be received by October 2, 2014, no scores will be accepted after this date. Scores are only accepted between June 1, 2014-October 2, 2014 and must be resent yearly if you are reapplying).
4. Complete VMCAS with electronic letters of recommendation
5. Complete Oregon State University supplemental application by October 2, 2014 at 12:00 PM PDT.
6. Pay online supplemental application fee of $50.00

## ENTRANCE REQUIREMENTS

All pre-requisites for OSU must be completed with a grade of C- or better.

*Is a Bachelor's Degree Required?* no

*Is this an International School?* yes

## ESTIMATED TUITION

*Estimated Tuition Resident:* $21,319

*Estimated Tuition Contract:* $21,319 plus additional $4000 per year scholarship

*Estimated Tuition Non-Resident:* $41,200

## PREREQUISITES FOR ADMISSION

| Course Description | Number of Hours/Credits | Necessity |
|---|---|---|
| General Biology I | 3 | Required |
| General Biology II | 3 | Required |
| Upper Division Biology | 4 | Required |
| Physics I | 4 | Required |
| Physics II | 4 | Required |
| General Chemistry I w/ Lab | 4 | Required |
| General Chemistry II w/ Lab | 4 | Required |
| Organic Chemistry I | 3 | Required |
| Biochemistry I | 4 | Required |
| Genetics | 3 | Required |
| Calculus or Algebra & Trig | 4 | Required |
| Statistics | 3 | Required |
| Physiology (Human or Animal) | 3 | Required |
| English | 4 | Required |
| Humanities or Social Sciences | 8 | Required |
| Public Speaking | 3 | Required |

## AVAILABLE SEATS

*Resident:* 40

*Contract:* 16

*Non-Resident:* 16

## TEST REQUIREMENTS

GRE general test

*VMCAS Participation:* full

*Accepts International Students?* yes

## ADDITIONAL INFORMATION

Conversion for quarter credits of our pre-requisites is available on our website.

*Application Deadline:* 10/2/2014

# UNIVERSITY OF PENNSYLVANIA

Email Address: admissions@vet.upenn.edu
Website: http://www.vet.upenn.edu

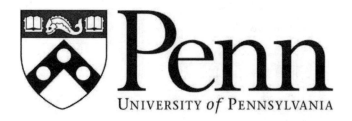

## SCHOOL DESCRIPTION

The University of Pennsylvania is located in West Philadelphia. Philadelphia is a city with a strong cultural heritage. Independence National Park includes 1 square mile of historic Philadelphia next to the Delaware River. Included are Independence Hall, the Liberty Bell, and many fine examples of colonial architecture. Philadelphia also offers theaters, museums, sports, and outdoor recreation. The Philadelphia Zoo, first in the nation, houses more than 1,600 mammals, birds, reptiles, and amphibians.

The School of Veterinary Medicine enjoys a close relationship with the zoo. The School of Veterinary Medicine was founded in 1884 and includes a hospital for small animals, classrooms, and research facilities in the city. The large-animal hospital and research facilities are located at the New Bolton Center, an 800-acre farm 40 miles west of Philadelphia. The first 2 years are spent on the main campus. Part of the third year may be spent at the New Bolton Center, and the fourth year is spent in rotation and on electives at varying campus locations. Off-campus electives are frequently permitted.

> The School of Veterinary Medicine enjoys a close relationship with the Philadelphia zoo, first in the nation.

## APPLICATION INFORMATION

For specific application information (availability, deadlines, fees, and VMCAS participation), please refer to the contact information listed above.

*Residency implications:* priority is given to Pennsylvania residents. The number of nonresident places is usually about 80, including international applicants.

*2012-2013 admissions summary for the class of 2017:*

|  | Number of Applicants | Number of Entrants |
|---|---|---|
| Resident | 243 | 45 |
| Non-Resident | 1,290 | 78 |
| Total | 1,533 | 123 |

## SUMMARY OF ADMISSION PROCEDURES

*Timetable*

*VMCAS application deadline:* Tuesday, October 2, 2014 at 1:00 PM Eastern Time

*Supplemental application and fee deadline:* October 2

*Date interviews are held:* Fridays from early January until completion

*Date acceptances mailed:* within 14 days after interview

*School begins:* early September

*Deposit (to hold place in class):* $500.00

*Deferments:* are considered on an individual basis.

## EVALUATION CRITERIA

The seats are filled through a 2-part admission procedure, which includes a file review and personal interviews.

Grades

Test scores

Animal/veterinary experience

## PREREQUISITES FOR ADMISSION

| Course Description | Number of Hours/Credits | Necessity |
| --- | --- | --- |
| English (including composition) | 6 | Required |
| Physics (with Lab) | 8 | Required |
| Chemistry - General (with at least 1 lab) | 8 | Required |
| Chemistry - Organic | 4 | Required |
| Biology or Zoology (covering basic genetics & cell bio) | 9 | Required |
| Biochem | 3 | Required |
| Microbiology | 3 | Required |
| Social sciences or humanities | 6 | Required |
| Calculus & Math Statistics (or biostats) | 6 | Required |
| Electives | 37 | Required |

Interview

References

Essay

English skills (TOEFL)

*File review:* files are reviewed in January by members of the admissions committee (including an alumni member), and decisions are made on whether or not to offer an interview.

*Personal interviews:* interviews are held on Fridays from early January until the class is filled. The number of interviews granted equals 1.5 to 2 times the number of seats available.

*Two personal interviews are conducted:* a formal interview with 2 faculty members (including an alumni member) of the committee, and an informal interview with student committee members. Although students do not vote on acceptance, they have a significant part in the meeting following interviews.

### ENTRANCE REQUIREMENTS

*Required undergraduate GPA:* no specific GPA. Applicants are evaluated comparatively. The mean cumulative GPA of the class admitted in 2013 was 3.64.

*AP credit policy:* must appear on official college transcripts and count toward degree.

*Course completion deadline:* All prerequisite courses must be completed by the end of the summer term of the year in which admission is sought.

### ADDITIONAL REQUIREMENTS/CONSIDERATIONS

*Animal/veterinary work experience:* experience working with animals, direct veterinary work, or research experience is desired. Approximately 500-600 hours is recommended. Experience should be sufficient to convince the admissions committee of motivation, interest, and understanding.

*Recommendations/evaluations:* 3 required, one from an academic science source; and one from a veterinarian. The third is the choice of the applicant.

*Extracurricular/community service activities:* additional activities in this category can provide information important to the admissions committee.

*Leadership:* evidence of leadership abilities is desirable.

*Is a Bachelor's Degree Required?* no

*Is this an International School?* no

### ESTIMATED TUITION

*Estimated Tuition Resident:* $39,866.00

*Estimated Tuition Contract:* Not Applicable

*Estimated Tuition Non-Resident:* $49,836.00

### AVAILABLE SEATS

*Resident:* 40

*Contract:* Not Applicable

*Non-Resident:* 80

## TEST REQUIREMENTS

*Standardized examinations:* Graduate Record Examination (GRE), general test, is required; the GRE Code for Pennvet is 2775. Test scores should be received no later than November 1.

*VMCAS Participation:* full

*Accepts International Students?* yes

## ADDITIONAL INFORMATION

*Dual-Degree Programs:* Combined VMD-graduate degree programs are available.

*Summer Program:* Penn Vet offers a summer program for high school and college students. The Veterinary Exploration Through Science (VETS) program, now in its fifth year is a day program of one-week sessions designed for those who want a close-up look at veterinary medicine. For additional information, please visit our website at www.vet.upenn.edu/education/admissions/summer-vets-program or call 215-898-5434.

*Application Deadline:* 10/2/2014

# FOURTH-YEAR PROFILE: JENNY SOWELL

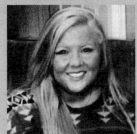

**What has been your favorite thing about attending veterinary school so far?**
My favorite thing about veterinary school has been getting to further my knowledge and exposure to an area that I am passionate about. Mississippi State University College of Veterinary Medicine has done an excellent job to ensure that its students are well-equipped for the field of veterinary medicine. I love the two-phase curriculum that we use and how we are able to customize our fourth year in order to expose ourselves to areas that we enjoy or want to improve in.

**What advice do you have for prospective veterinary school applicants?**
Have an open mind about the career. There are so many directions to go in this field now, especially with the growth in the public health aspect. I think it is wonderful to have a keen interest in a particular area, but it is important to at least explore the other possible routes that exist for veterinarians.

**What do you plan on doing after graduating veterinary school?**
After graduation, I plan to find a job at a small or mixed animal practice in Mississippi. My husband is a high school agriculture teacher and loves his job. We hope to stay in our home state, as it is where our family lives and the place we are proud to call home.

**What extracurricular activities have you been involved in during veterinary school?**
I have served as class vice president for all four years. I have also been an MSU-CVM envoy, which is someone who gives tours of our school and talks to prospective students and school groups. I also served as the 2012 MSU-CVM open house student coordinator, which brings thousands of schoolchildren to tour our facility and participate in various fun activities. The following are clubs that I have been active in while in veterinary school: student chapter of Disaster Animal Response, Christian Veterinary Fellowship, American Association of Feline Practitioners, Wildlife Exotic Zoo Aquatic Avian Medicine Club, Surgery Club, Mississippi Animal Response Team, Merial Student Representative.

**What was the biggest challenge you faced during veterinary school?**
The biggest challenge has been prioritizing my studies. During our first two years of veterinary school, we would often have multiple exams in one week. I would find it difficult to devote enough study time to one exam, due to spending too much time on another. I was able to improve on as time went on.

**What advice do you have for other students who are currently in veterinary school?**
My advice to students is to "keep on keeping on." Though it does not seem like it at times, there is a light at the end. I also recommend getting to know your classmates. I have made lifelong friends, and I know that I will be able to call any of them should I need advice or support once I am out in practice. Take advantage of any externship opportunities, for they are wonderful tools to not only learn more, but may lead to a potential job offer.

**Why do you want to be a veterinarian?**
I want to be a veterinarian because it is where I feel that I am fulfilling my utmost potential. I can help people, help animals, and strengthen the bond that is so special. I have a great deal of passion for this field and have been fortunate enough to work with many veterinarians who have been wonderful mentors.

**Are you taking advantage of any scholarship, loans, or loan repayment programs?**
I have used federal loans to pay for veterinary school, but I have only used what I need for tuition. I have been fortunate to have a working spouse who has done a phenomenal job in supporting us these past four years. I have also received various scholarships while in school, with a couple of them assisting me with distant externship opportunities. As far as loan repayment programs, I plan to use the income-based repayment plan.

# PURDUE UNIVERSITY

Email Address: vetadmissions@purdue.edu
Website: http://www.vet.purdue.edu

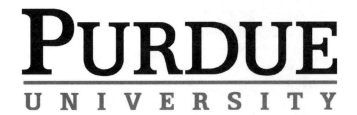

## SCHOOL DESCRIPTION

Purdue University is located in one of the largest metropolitan centers in northwestern Indiana. Greater Lafayette occupies a site on the Wabash River 65 miles northwest of Indianapolis and 126 miles southeast of Chicago. The combined population of the twin cities, Lafayette and West Lafayette, exceeds 100,000. The community offers an art museum, historical museum, 1,600 acres of public parks, and more than 60 churches of all major denominations.

> Purdue emphasizes the veterinary team approach, problem solving, and hands-on experiences.

Purdue ranks among the 25 largest colleges and universities in the nation. Students represent all 50 states and many foreign countries. Purdue University has the second highest enrollment of international students of any college in the United States. The Purdue University College of Veterinary Medicine strives to become the leading veterinary school for comprehensive education of the veterinary team and for discovery and engagement in selected areas of veterinary and comparative biomedical sciences. To better prepare individuals for veterinary medical careers in the twenty-first century, our curriculum emphasizes the veterinary team approach, problem solving, and hands-on experiences.

## APPLICATION INFORMATION

For specific application information, please refer to the contact information listed above. Purdue Veterinary Medicine requires a brief supplemental application. The application can be obtained at www.vet.purdue.edu/admissions. The deadline for submission is October 2, 2014.

Each veterinary class has 84 students. The class will be seated with approximately 50% residents and 50% nonresident students.

## SUMMARY OF ADMISSION PROCEDURES

*Timetable*

*VMCAS application deadline:* Thursday, October 2, 2014 1:00 PM Eastern Time

*Purdue Supplemental Application deadline:* October 2, 2014 1:00 PM Eastern Time

*Date interviews are held:* January

*Date acceptances mailed:* February

*Classes begin:* late August

*Deposit (to hold place in class):* $250.00 for residents; $1,000.00 for nonresidents. Deposit applied to tuition after matriculation.

*Deferments:* request for deferments will be considered on a case-by-case basis.

## EVALUATION CRITERIA

The admission process consists of:

A preliminary review based upon grade point indices, test scores, and prerequisite course completion

An in-depth review of selected applicants

A personal interview by invitation is required

% Weight

Grades, test scores, overall academic performance - 55% weight (including honors courses, study abroad)

| Course Description | Semesters | Necessity |
|---|---|---|
| Inorganic Chemistry with Lab I | 4 | Required |
| Inorganic Chemistry with Lab II | 4 | Required |
| Organic Chemistry with Lab I | 3 | Required |
| Organic Chemistry with Lab II | 3 | Required |
| Biochemistry (upperlevel) | 3 | Required |
| Biology with Lab I | 4 | Required |
| Biology with Lab II | 4 | Required |
| Genetics with Lab | 3 | Required |
| Microbiology with Lab | 4 | Required |
| Animal Nutrition | 3 | Required |
| Physics with Lab I | 4 | Required |
| Physics with Lab II | 4 | Required |
| Calculus | 3 | Required |
| Statistics | 3 | Required |
| English Composition | 3 | Required |
| Communication | 3 | Required |
| Humanities I | 3 | Required |
| Humanities II | 3 | Required |
| Humanities III | 3 | Required |

Animal, veterinary, research, and general work experiences, extracurricular activities, personal statement, overall presentation of application materials, honors and awards, references, and interview - 45% weight

## ENTRANCE REQUIREMENTS

*Required undergraduate GPA:* the mean cumulative GPA of the entering class in the fall of 2013 for resident students was 3.75 on a 4.00 scale and for non-resident students was 3.63 on a 4.00 scale. The minimum cumulative GPA required for consideration is 2.75 on a 4.00 scale.

*AP credit policy:* will be accepted if it appears on official college transcripts by subject area and is equivalent to the appropriate college-level coursework. Should your institution's official transcript not list the subject area, then you may submit an unofficial transcript with a letter explaining this and indicating which prerequisite courses are met by these credits.

*Is a Bachelor's Degree Required?* no

*Is this an International School?* no

## ESTIMATED TUITION

*Estimated Tuition Resident:* $19,418

*Estimated Tuition Contract:* n/a

*Estimated Tuition Non-Resident:* $44,246

## AVAILABLE SEATS

*Resident:* 42

*Contract:* 0

*Non-Resident:* 42

## TEST REQUIREMENTS

*Standardized examinations:* Purdue University will only accept scores of the revised GRE. Scores must be submitted by the October 2nd deadline. Use the Purdue University Grad School code of 1631.

*VMCAS Participation:* full

*Accepts International Students?* yes

## ADDITIONAL INFORMATION:

*Application Deadline:* 10/2/2014

# UNIVERSITY OF TENNESSEE

Email Address: dshepherd@utk.edu
Website: http://www.vet.utk.edu

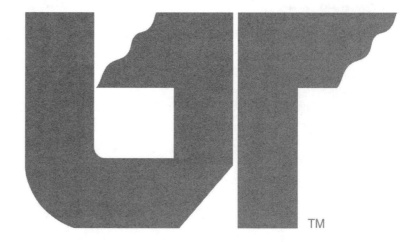

## SCHOOL DESCRIPTION

The University of Tennessee's College of Veterinary Medicine is located in Knoxville, a city of 185,000 situated in the Appalachian foothills of east central Tennessee. Only 45 minutes from the Great Smoky Mountains National Park and 3 hours from both Nashville and Atlanta, Knoxville offers many recreational and cultural opportunities, including a symphony orchestra, an opera company, and several fine theaters. The climate in Knoxville is moderate with distinct seasons.

> The Knoxville campus of the University of Tennessee has about 21,300 undergraduate and 6,200 graduate students.

The 550-acre Knoxville campus of the University of Tennessee has about 21,300 undergraduate and 6,200 graduate students. The modern Clyde M. York Veterinary Medicine Building, housing the teaching and research facilities, the Veterinary Medical Center, including the W.W. Armistead Veterinary Teaching Hospital, and Agriculture-Veterinary Medicine Library, faces the Tennessee River on the university's Agricultural Campus.

The curriculum of the College of Veterinary Medicine is a 9-semester, 4-year program. Development of a strong basic science education is emphasized in the first year. The second and third years emphasize the study of diseases, their causes, diagnosis, treatment, and prevention. Innovative features of the first three years of the curriculum include 6 weeks of student-centered small-group applied-learning exercises in semesters 1-5; 3 weeks of dedicated clinical experiences in the Veterinary Medical Center in semesters 3-5; and

elective course opportunities in semesters 4-9 that allow students to focus on specific educational/ career goals. In the fourth year (final 3 semesters), students participate exclusively in clinical rotations (27 weeks of core rotations and 23 weeks of elective rotations) in the Veterinary Medical Center and in required off-campus externships. The college has unique programs in zoo, avian, and exotic animal medicine and surgery, cancer diagnosis and therapy, minimally invasive surgery (laser lithotripsy, endoscopy, otoscopy), and rehabilitation/physical therapy.

## APPLICATION INFORMATION

For specific application information (availability, deadlines, fees, and VMCAS participation), please refer to the contact information listed above. We admit approximately 85 applicants each year. Priority is given to Tennessee residents (60 of the 85 seats are for Tennessee residents). Twenty-five highly qualified non-residents are admitted each year.

*Residency implications:* Tennessee has no contractual agreements and does accept nonresident applications. Tennessee accepts applications only from United States citizens and permanent residents of the United States. International applications are not considered.

## SUMMARY OF ADMISSION PROCEDURES

*Timetable*

*VMCAS application deadline:* October 1, 2014, 1:00 PM Eastern Time

GRE scores must be received by the College no later than October 1, 2014

*Date interviews are held:* January 5, 6, and 10, 2015

*Date acceptances mailed:* no later than January 30, 2015

*Applicant's response date:* April 15, 2015

*School begins:* late August 2015

*Deposit (to hold place in class):* none required.

*Deferments:* are considered on a case-by-case basis.

## EVALUATION CRITERIA

The admission procedure consists of a 3-phased review process (i.e., academic review, packet review, and interview). Each section weighted equally in the final applicant score. The initial academic review determines which applicants will move forward to a packet review. The combined academic review and packet review determines selection of the applicant interview pool.

*Initial academic file review includes:*
Academic performance and grade point average
GRE Test scores
Prerequisite completion
VMCAS and Supplemental Application information
VMCAS Disadvantaged/Hardship statement

*Holistic packet review:*
Rigor of educational program
Personal Statement
References (3-6 required)
Evidence of logical preparation for this career
Veterinary and Animal Experience
Extracurricular activities/community service
Leadership and diversity
Disadvantaged/Hardship factors

*Interview:*
Personal Statement
Communication skills
Motivation
Animal/veterinary experience
Understanding of the profession
Personal interests and qualities
Professionalism

## ENTRANCE REQUIREMENTS

*Required undergraduate GPA:* for nonresident applicants, the minimum acceptable cumulative GPA is 3.20 on a 4.00 scale. At time of acceptance, the mean GPA of the class entering in fall of 2013 was 3.66.

*AP credit policy:* must appear on official college transcripts and be equivalent to the appropriate college-level coursework.

*Course completion deadline:* prerequisite courses must be completed with a grade of C or better by the end of the spring term prior to entry.

*Is a Bachelor's Degree Required?* no

*Is this an International School?* no

## ESTIMATED TUITION

*Estimated Tuition Resident:* $24,022

*Estimated Tuition Contract:* $0

*Estimated Tuition Non-Resident:* $52,122

## AVAILABLE SEATS

*Resident:* 60

*Contract:* 0

*Non-Resident:* 25

## TEST REQUIREMENTS

*Standardized examinations:* Graduate Record Exam (GRE), General Test (Verbal, Quantitative, and Analytical) is required, and scores must be received by October 1, 2014.

*VMCAS Participation:* full

*Accepts International Students?* no

## ADDITIONAL INFORMATION

*Additional requirements and considerations:*
    Animal/veterinary work experience
    3 letters of recommendation are required but no more than 6 letters will be accepted
    Extracurricular and/community service activities
    Leadership skills
    Autobiographical essay (personal statement)
    A Supplemental Application is required and an optional Disadvantages Declaration and can be found at: http://www.utk.edu/admissions/supplemental.php

*Parallel Degree Program*

The College, in partnership with the College of Education, Health and Human Sciences, offeres an option for veterinary students (and graduate veterinarians) to earn the MPH degree with a concentration in Veterinairy Public Health.

Contact the College of Veterinary Medicine, Dr. Marcy Souza at msouza@utk.edu for additional information.

# TEXAS A&M UNIVERSITY

Texas A&M University
College of Veterinary Medicine & Biomedical Sciences
Email Address: studentadmissions@cvm.tamu.edu
Website: http://vetmed.tamu.edu

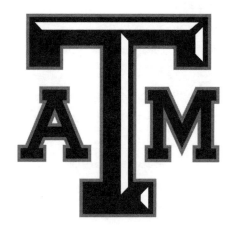

## SCHOOL DESCRIPTION

The university is located adjacent to the cities of Bryan and College Station. The two cities have a combined population of about 100,000. The student population at Texas A & M is more than 58,000. The College of Veterinary Medicine is one of the 10 original veterinary teaching institutions that existed in the United States prior to World War II.

The College provides an integrated professional curriculum that prepares graduates with a firm foundation in the basic sciences, a broad comparative medicine knowledge base, and the clinical and personal skills to be leaders in the many career fields of veterinary medicine. Professional students are given the opportunity to gain additional education and training in their personal career paths.

> The College of Veterinary Medicine is one of the 10 original teaching institutions that existed in the US prior to World War II.

Becoming a veterinarian requires much dedication and diligent study. The veterinary medical student is required to meet a high level of performance. The demands on students' time and effort are considerable, but the rewards and career satisfaction are personal achievements that make significant contributions to our society.

## APPLICATION INFORMATION

For specific application information (availability, deadlines and fees), please refer to the contact information listed above.

*Residency implications:* Texas has no contractual agreements with other states. Applicants from other states who have outstanding credentials will be considered. Texas seats 122 residents and up to 10 non-resident applicants per year. In the event that not all 10 non-resident positions are filled, these positions will then be filled with Texas alternates. Successful candidates who are awarded competitive university-based scholarships may attend at resident tuition rate.

## SUMMARY OF ADMISSION PROCEDURES

*Timetable*

*Application deadline:* October 1

*Date interviews are held:* mid-January

*Date acceptances mailed:* mid-March

*School begins:* late August

*Deposit (to hold place in class):* none required.

*Deferments:* requests for deferments will be considered on a case-by-case basis.

## EVALUATION CRITERIA

Academic performance

Test scores

Interview

Personal statement

Evaluations (3 evaluations are required. 1 evaluation must be from a veterinarian with whom you have worked with. No letters of support/recommendation are needed)

## PREREQUISITES FOR ADMISSION

| Course Description | Number of Hours/Credits | Necessity |
|---|---|---|
| General Biology with lab | 4 | Required |
| General Microbiology with lab | 4 | Required |
| Genetics | 3 | Required |
| Animal Nutrition or Feeds & Feeding | 3 | Required |
| Inorganic Chemistry I & II with lab | 8 | Required |
| Organic Chemistry I & II with lab | 8 | Required |
| Biochemistry (lecture hours only) | 5 | Required |
| Statistics (upper level) | 3 | Required |
| Physics I & II with lab | 8 | Required |
| Composition & Rhetoric | 3 | Required |
| Introduction to Psychology | 3 | Required |
| Technical Writing | 3 | Required |
| Speech Communication | 3 | Required |

Semester course load and post-academic challenge

Leadership and experience

Entrance Requirements

*Required undergraduate GPA:* the minimum overall GPA required is 2.90 on a 4.00 scale or 3.10 for the last 45 semester credits. The mean of the most recent entering class was 3.65.

*AP credit policy:* AP credit is accepted as fulfilling selected prerequisites; credit must be reflected on the official undergraduate transcript.

*Is a Bachelor's Degree Required?* no

*Is this an International School?* no

### ESTIMATED TUITION

*Estimated Tuition Resident:* $20,348

*Estimated Tuition Contract:* $0

*Estimated Tuition Non-Resident:* $31,148

### AVAILABLE SEATS

*Resident:* 122

*Contract:* 0

*Non-Resident:* 10

### TEST REQUIREMENTS

Standardized examinations: Graduate Record Examination (GRE), general test, is required. Beginning August 1, 2011, the College of Veterinary Medicine will require the new version of the GRE examination.

*VMCAS Participation:* non-vmcas

*Accepts International Students?* no

### ADDITIONAL INFORMATION

*Application Deadline:* 10/1/2014

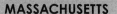

# TUFTS UNIVERSITY

Email Address: vetadmissions@tufts.edu
Website: http://www.tufts.edu/vet/

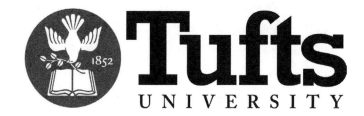

## SCHOOL DESCRIPTION

Tufts University is located near Boston, where athletic and cultural activities abound. The Cummings School of Veterinary Medicine provides an exciting biomedical environment for the study of cutting-edge veterinary medicine. Signature programs include: wildlife and conservation medicine, international veterinary medicine, animal welfare, ethics and policy, and accelerated clinical excellence. Issues related to the ethical dimensions of veterinary medicine, including animal welfare, are an integral aspect of the curriculum. Hands-on learning begins in the first year and continues throughout the curriculum. Many opportunities exist outside of formal courses for hands-on work in hospitals and research laboratories. The Hospital for Large Animals, Foster Hospital for Small Animals, the Ambulatory Service, the Wildlife Clinic, and Tufts at Tech provide a rich mixture of learning opportunities with horses, cats, dogs, cattle, sheep, goats, and native wildlife. Our large caseload, ranked among the top three schools in the country, provides an exciting and challenging education for students.

> Many opportunities exist outside of formal courses for hands-on work in hospitals and research laboratories.

## APPLICATION INFORMATION

For specific application information (availability, deadlines, fees, and VMCAS participation), please refer to the contact information listed above.

*Residency implications:* Massachusetts residents make up about one-third of each class. All other applicants considered for the remaining spaces.

## SUMMARY OF ADMISSION PROCEDURES

*Timetable*

*Application deadline:* November 1

*Date interviews are held:* December, January, February

*Date acceptances mailed:* March

*School begins:* late August

*Deposit (to hold place in class):* $500.00

*Deferments:* requests for deferment are handled on a case-by-case basis.

## EVALUATION CRITERIA

Tufts' admission procedure consists of a review of the application and an interview of selected applicants.

## ENTRANCE REQUIREMENTS

Required undergraduate GPA: no minimum GPA required. The mean GPA for the Class of 2017 was 3.65.

*AP credit policy:* must appear on official college transcripts and be equivalent to the appropriate college-level coursework.

*Is a Bachelor's Degree Required?* no

*Is this an International School?* no

## PREREQUISITES FOR ADMISSION

| Course Description | Number of Hours/Credits | Necessity |
|---|:---:|:---:|
| Biology with laboratory | 8 | Required |
| Chemistry with laboratory | 8 | Required |
| Organic chemistry with laboratory | 8 | Required |
| Biochemistry | 3 | Required |
| Physics | 3 | Required |
| Genetics* | 3 | Required |
| Mathematics/Statistics | 6 | Required |
| English/Speech | 6 | Required |
| Humanities and Fine Arts | 6 | Required |
| Social and Behavioral Sciences | 6 | Required |

* unless included in biology

## ESTIMATED TUITION

*Estimated Tuition Resident:* $41,940

*Estimated Tuition Contract:* $0

*Estimated Tuition Non-Resident:* $46,120

## AVAILABLE SEATS

*Resident:* 32

*Contract:* 0

*Non-Resident:* 66

## TEST REQUIREMENTS

*Standardized examinations:* Graduate Record Examinations (GRE), general test, is required. The most recent acceptable test date for applicants to the class of 2019 is October 31, 2014. Scores are valid for five years. The mean GRE scores for the Class of 2017 were: Verbal 162, Quantitative 159, and Analytical Writing 4.5.

*VMCAS Participation:* non-VMCAS

*Accepts International Students?* yes

## ADDITIONAL INFORMATION

*Application Deadline:* 11/1/2014

# TUSKEGEE UNIVERSITY*

Office of Veterinary Admissions and Recruitment
Tuskegee University School of Veterinary Medicine
Tuskegee, AL 36088
Telephone: (334) 727-8460
Website: www.onemedicine.tuskegee.edu

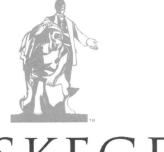

## TUSKEGEE
### UNIVERSITY

## SCHOOL DESCRIPTION

Tuskegee University School of Veterinary Medicine is located in Tuskegee, Alabama, a city of about 13,000. Tuskegee is 40 miles east of the state of Alabama, Capitol city, Montgomery, and twenty miles west of the city of Auburn. It is also within easy driving distance to the cities of Birmingham, Alabama and Atlanta, Georgia. Summers are hot with moderate to mild humidity, and winters are moderate. Its recreational facilities, lakes, and parks can be enjoyed throughout the year-round.

> The University stresses the need to educate the whole person, that is, the hand and the heart as well as the mind.

Over the past 125 years and still today, since it was founded by Booker T. Washington in 1881, Tuskegee University (HBCU) has become one of our nation's most outstanding institutions of higher learning. While it focuses on helping to develop human resources primarily within the African-American community, it is open to all.

Tuskegee's mission has always been to provide service to people in addition to education. The University stresses the need to educate the whole person, that is, the hand and the heart as well as the mind. Tuskegee enrolls more than 3,000 students and employs approximately 900 faculty and support personnel. Physical facilities include more than 5,000 acres of forestry and a campus consisting of more than 100 major buildings and structures. Total land, forestry, and facilities are valued in excess of $500 million. The campus has also been declared a historical site by the United States Department of the Interior.

Historically, Tuskegee University School of Veterinary Medicine (TUSVM) was established in 1945 for the training of African-Americans during a time when few had the opportunity to study veterinary medicine because of segregation and other racial impediments.

In 1945, the United States had only 10 schools of veterinary medicine and it is estimated that fewer than five African Americans were located in the southern states. TUSVM graduated its first class of fully qualified veterinarians in 1949. Since then, it has graduated more than 70% of the African-American veterinarians in the United States.

Today, TUSVM is one of 28 Schools/Colleges of Veterinary Medicine in the United States. However, it is the only one in the U.S. that is fully integrated, serving African-Americans, Caucasian students, Hispanics, Asians, Native Americans and international students. TUSVM is the most racially, 125 ethnically, and culturally diverse school of veterinary medicine in North America.

Also, TUSVM's graduates have excelled in private clinical practice, in public practice such as in the government, in the military, and in corporations such as the pharmaceutical industry. They hold key leadership positions in the government, military, academia, and in the international arena.

Tuskegee University School of Veterinary Medicine is fully accredited by the American Veterinary Medical Association (AVMA) and its Veterinary Teaching Hospital is accredited by the American Animal Hospital Association (AAHA).

*These pages are for last year's admissions cycle. For updated information, please visit: www.onemedicine.tuskegee.edu

## PREREQUISITES FOR ADMISSION

### Courses and Requirements in Semester Hours

| | |
|---|---|
| I. English or Written Composition | 6 |
| II. Mathematics | 6 |
| III. Social Sciences / Humanities | 6 |
| IV. Liberal Arts | 6 |
| | 24 |
| VI. Biological & Physical Sciences | |
| Advance Biology (300 Level or Above)** | 9 |
| Biochemistry w/Lab | 4 |
| Advance Biology Elective | 8 |
| Organic Chemistry w/Lab | 4 |
| Physics w/Lab | 8 |
| | 33 |
| VI. Animal Science*** | |
| Introduction to Animal Science | 3 |
| Animal Nutrition | 3 |
| | 6 |
| **Total Semester Hours** | 63 |

** Advanced biology courses, e.g., anatomy, physiology, ecology, immunology, zoology, microbiology, genetics, toxicology, and histology
*** Applicants who do not include animal science courses in their Pre-Professional studies may be admitted at the discretion of the Admissions Committee, if they fulfilled all other requirements. However, these courses must be completed prior to attaining third-year status in the Tuskegee University School of Veterinary Medicine. From year 2017 forward all animal science courses have to be completed before enrollment at the veterinary school.

## APPLICATION INFORMATION

Application Fee: $205.00 TUSVM requires a processing fee to develop and maintain each applicant's computerized database. Send Application fee directly to Tuskegee University School of Veterinary Medicine-Office of Admissions and Recruitment.

For specific application information (availability, deadlines, fees, and VMCAS), please refer to the contact information listed above, or visit the online application process at: www.onemedicine.tuskegee.edu.

*Residency implications:* applications are accepted with special consideration given to Alabama residents and those who have residency in the following contract states, Kentucky, South Carolina, and Arkansas.

Number of resident seats, non-resident seat: none - TUSVM maintains "open access" and selection for seats.

International applications will be considered for admissions into TUSVM

## PREREQUISITES FOR ADMISSION

The Tuskegee University School of Veterinary Medicine's professional curriculum is a rigorous four-year program. Therefore applicant's final grade for each

required course must be a "C" or better. Students are required to take the General Aptitude portion of the Graduate Record Examination (GRE). Additionally, there is a mandatory interview with the TUSVM Admissions Committee before acceptance into the school is granted.

*GPA:* the cumulative and science GPA requirement is 2.7 on a 4.00 scale.

*Course completion deadline:* prerequisite courses must be completed by end of May.

*Standardized examinations:* Graduate Record Examination (GRE) of which must be taken within three years of application, is required. Must be completed by October 1. Request GRE Test Scores results by November 1.

## SUMMARY OF ADMISSION PROCEDURE

*Timetable*

*Application deadline:* October 2

*Date interviews are held:* January–February

*Date acceptances mailed:* April 15

*School begins:* mid-August

*Deferments:* one-year deferments are considered on a case-by-case basis.

## EVALUATION CRITERIA

The following items are taken into consideration: academic record, academic trends, letters of recommendation, work experience, and test scores.

|  | % weight |
|---|---|
| Grades | 68 |
| Test scores | 8 |
| Animal/veterinary experience | 6 |
| Interview | 15 |
| References |  |
|    Science Professors | 2 |
|    Veterinarian | 1 |
| Essay (Handwritten, see application) |  |

*Number of available seats:* Approximately 65-70

## EXPENSES FOR THE 2012–2013 ACADEMIC YEAR

*Tuition and fees*

*In state:* $10,860.00 per semester

*Out of state:* $18,135.00 per semester

*Technology fee:* $200.00

*I.D. fee:* $30.00

*Application Fee:* $205.00

If admitted, additional fees and expenses are required.

## DUAL-DEGREE PROGRAMS

Combined DVM–Graduate Degree Programs are available: PhD in Integrative Biosciences, PhD Interdisciplinary Pathobiology, Master of Science Veterinary Science, Master of Science Tropical Animal Health, Master of Public Health and Master of Science in Public Health

# FIRST-YEAR PROFILE: LAUREL A. DOVE

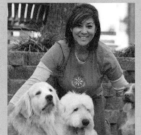

### Why do you want to be a veterinarian?
Helping others is truly was drives me, and I can't think of a better way than to help animals in need. I believe that the animal-human bond is so important, and by helping animals, I believe this is also helping humans.

### What are your short-term and long-term goals?
Short term, I would like to work in a mixed animal clinic. Long term, I would like to continue working in a mixed animal clinic, while incorporating shelter animal assistance.

### What did you do as an applicant to prepare for veterinary school?
Having served in the military, I completed my bachelor's degree, and I feel that I gained a lot of leadership and communication skills. After retiring, I volunteered at a veterinary clinic, worked full time at a veterinary clinic, and began taking classes to become a licensed vet tech. After realizing my goal was truly to become a veterinarian, I began pursuing my prerequisites for veterinary school. I volunteered for courses and opportunities that gave me exposure to anything related to the veterinary field.

### What advice would you give to applicants or those considering veterinary school?
No matter what class you are taking, learn it as though you will use it in veterinary school and as a practicing veterinarian. I have been amazed at how much of my undergraduate classes apply to what I have learned in vet school. I have found that even information from classes that did not seem applicable to veterinary medicine are referenced or will be very helpful in my future veterinary career.

### What helped make the transition to veterinary school easier?
Being able to recall information from undergraduate classes and having experience in the military helped me to transition.

### What is your advice on financial aid?
I served and retired from the military, so I am receiving education benefits that cover approximately half of the costs of attending veterinary school.

### What are you most excited about learning in veterinary school?
I'd like to say everything, but if I have to narrow it down, I would say that when I learn about a condition that I saw in a patient during my time as a technician, I get very excited to understand that condition, how it might have manifested, and how it can possibly be treated.

### What advice do you have for students who are considering applying to veterinary school?
Like many aspiring veterinarians, I have always had an affinity for caring for animals of all kinds. While driving down a dusty road as a young girl in the Middle East, my parents asked me what I wanted to be when I grew up. I told them that I didn't know, and they said that I would be a great veterinarian. I didn't even know what a veterinarian was, but when they told me, it was then that I began my lifelong dream of veterinary medicine.

# VIRGINIA-MARYLAND REGIONAL COLLEGE OF VETERINARY MEDICINE

Email Address: dvmadmit@vt.edu
Website: http://www.becomeavet.vetmed.vt.edu/

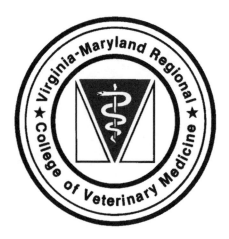

## SCHOOL DESCRIPTION

The Virginia-Maryland Regional College of Veterinary Medicine is situated on 3 distinct campuses. The main campus is at Virginia Tech in Blacksburg, Virginia, a community with a population of about 40,000 situated on a high plateau in southwestern Virginia between the Blue Ridge and Allegheny Mountains. Its residents enjoy a wide range of educational, social, recreational, and cultural opportunities. In addition to the Blacksburg campus, the Equine Medical Center campus is in Leesburg, Virginia, and the University of Maryland is at College Park.

> The College offers students the opportunity to receive advanced training to conduct research in basic or clinical disciplines.

In recognition of a need for veterinarians trained in both basic and clinical sciences, the college offers students the opportunity to participate in graduate studies and receive appropriate advanced training to conduct research in basic or clinical disciplines. Nearly 25 percent of the nation's veterinarians work in areas other than private practice, such as government and corporate veterinary medicine. Through the assistance of a grant from the Pew Charitable Trusts, the college has established the Center for Public and Corporate Veterinary Medicine, which is a national resource for training veterinarians for the wide variety of careers in this area of the profession.

## APPLICATION INFORMATION

For specific application information (availability, deadlines, fees, and VMCAS participation), please refer to our website at: http://www.becomeavet.vetmed.vt.edu/

*Residency implications:* 50 positions are reserved for Virginia residents, and 30 positions for Maryland residents. Up to 40 additional positions may be filled by nonresidents, 6 of those reserved for WV residents.

## SUMMARY OF ADMISSION PROCEDURES

*Timetable*

*Supplemental application deadline:* October 2, 2014 (The supplemental application can be accessed at: http://www.becomeavet.vetmed.vt.edu/howto/steps_to_apply)

*Date interviews are held:* TBD

*Date acceptances mailed:* early March

*School begins:* mid-August

*Deposit (to hold place in class):* $400 for residents and non-residents

*Deferments:* case-by-case basis if a candidate has extenuating circumstances beyond his or her control.

## EVALUATION CRITERIA

The admission procedure is comprised of an initial screening of applicants, review of the application portfolios, and interviews of selected applicants.

*Evaluation*

70%: Academics: cumulative GPA, required science GPA, last 45 semester hour GPA, GRE aptitude

**PREREQUISITES FOR ADMISSION**

| Course Description | Number of Hours/Credits | Necessity |
|---|---|---|
| General Biology | 8 | Required |
| Organic Chemistry | 8 | Required |
| General or Introductory Physics | 8 | Required |
| Biochemistry | 3 | Required |
| Humanities/Social Sciences | 6 | Required |
| Math: algebra, geometry, trigonometry, calculus, or statistics | 6 | Required |
| English (3 semester hours must be English composition or a writing-intensive designated course) | 6 | Required |

30%: Non-Academics: related animal experience, veterinary experience; research, industrial, and biomedical experiences; references; and overall application portfolio review

Interviews

Top candidates ranked on the above criteria will be invited for interviews. Admission offers will be based on interview results.

### ENTRANCE REQUIREMENTS

Students must earn a "C" or better in all required courses.

Science courses taken 7 or more years ago may be repeated or substituted with higher-level courses with the written consent of the admissions committee.

*Required undergraduate GPA:* to be considered for admission, applicants must have a cumulative GPA of at least 2.80 on a 4.00 scale upon completion of a minimum of 2 academic years of full-time study (60 semester/90 quarter hours) at an accredited college or university. Alternatively, a 3.30 GPA in the last 2 years (60 semester hours) will qualify a student who does not have a 2.80 GPA overall. All courses taken during this 2-year period must be junior or senior level. The mean GPA of those accepted into the class of 2016 was 3.5.

Advanced placement credit for 1 semester of English will be accepted if the additional required hours are composition or technical writing and are taken at a college or university.

Advanced placement credit or credit by examination for preveterinary course requirements will be accepted. Those credits must appear on the applicant's college transcript. Advanced placement credits will not be cal-

culated in grade point averages and no grade assigned. No course substitutions will be allowed for AP credit or credit by examination.

*Course completion deadline:* required courses must be completed by the end of the spring term of the year in which matriculation occurs.

*Standardized examinations:* Graduate Record Examination (GRE) scores must be received by November 1, 2014. It is advised that the test be taken by the first week of October.

*Letters of recommendation:* Three electronic evaluations/letters of recommendation are required.

### ADDITIONAL REQUIREMENTS AND CONSIDERATIONS

Maturity and a broad cultural perspective

Motivation and dedication to a career in veterinary medicine

Evidence of potential, and appreciation of the career opportunities for veterinarians, as indicated by:
1. Clinical veterinary experience (private practice)
2. Animal experience in addition to time spent working with a veterinarian
3. Biomedical/research experience (such as working with veterinarians or other biomedically trained individuals in health care, government, research laboratories, industrial, or corporate settings.)
4. Extramural activities, achievements, honors
5. Communication skills
6. References

*Is a Bachelor's Degree Required?* no

*Is this an International School?* no

## ESTIMATED TUITION

*Estimated Tuition Resident:* $21,796 per year

*Estimated Tuition Non-Resident:* $47,458 per year

## AVAILABLE SEATS

*Resident:* 80

*Contract:* 6

*Non-Resident:* 34

## TEST REQUIREMENTS

Graduate Record Examination (GRE) scores must be received by November 1, 2014. It is advised that the test be taken by the first week of October.

*VMCAS Participation:* full

*Accepts International Students?* yes

## ADDITIONAL INFORMATION

*Application Deadline:* 10/2/2014

# PRE-VETERINARIAN PROFILE: SASKIA FREDERICK

**YEAR OF GRADUATION**
2015

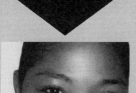

### What type of veterinary medicine are you interested in pursuing?
I am interested in pursuing large animal medicine or shelter medicine (I am hoping to make a decision by next year after a few more experiences in both areas).

### What did you major in during undergrad?
I have a BA in Political Science/Pre-law, and I am working to complete an AS/BS in Veterinary Technology with vet school prerequisites.

### What are your short-term and long-term goals?
My short-term goals are to complete my undergraduate degree and take the vet tech licensing exam. I also want to pursue my master's degree in Public Health during fall 2014. Long-term goals include working as a DVM for the United Nations.

### What are you doing as an applicant/pre-vet to prepare for veterinary school?
I am taking the required classes, fulfilling professorships/animal experiences hours at clinics and hospitals.

### What extracurricular activities are you involved in currently?
I am an upper class senator on the Student Government Association, the president of the Vet Tech club, vice president of the Future DVM club, and the president of the Intervarsity Christian Fellowship Club. Through these clubs I participate in volunteering on campus and in the community for different issues.

### How old were you when you first became interested in being a veterinarian?
I was five when I realized that I wanted to work with animals, but I was thirteen when I became first interested in being a veterinarian. One of our sows attempted to cannibalize her young after birth and my parents were about to euthanize the piglets. I sneaked about five of them to my bedroom and started treating them. They all survived, including the piglet who'd lost and entire hind limb (he walked on the bone of it). I realized then that this was what I wanted to do with my life.

### Have you shadowed or worked with any veterinarians in preparation to apply to vet school?
This past summer I interned for the first time at a small animal hospital. Initially, it was supposed to be primarily a shadow experience. My very first day I observed (and helped to prep for) a nephrectomy. It was my first time encountering bilateral neurosis as I was still a first-year student. During my time there the doctors took the time out to teach me, for which I was very grateful. I learned surgical practices and bandaging techniques before I even took these classes. I also encountered septicemia for the first time, a case I will never forget! It was a very hands-on experience (some days I actually got homework). This experience cemented in my mind that this was truly what I want to do.

### What characteristics are you looking for in a veterinary school?
Small classroom size, accessibility to lecturers, field /study abroad opportunities, AVMA accreditation, and a diverse student body are some of the most important characteristics I am looking for.

### What advice do you have for students who are considering applying to veterinary school?
Have back-up plans, build a portfolio of diverse experiences and qualifications, have an idea of the type of medicine that you're interested in, and research the schools—even visit a few. Network, network, network!

# WASHINGTON STATE UNIVERSITY

Email Address: admissions@vetmed.wsu.edu
Website: www.vetmed.wsu.edu/ProspectiveStudents

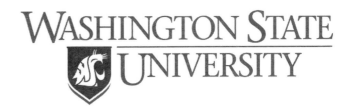

## SCHOOL DESCRIPTION

The Washington-Idaho-Montana-Utah (WIMU) regional program in veterinary medicine is a partnership between the Washington State University College of Veterinary Medicine, University of Idaho Department of Animal and Veterinary Science, Montana State University, and Utah State University School of Veterinary Medicine. The WSU College of Veterinary Medicine is also a partner with the Western Interstate Commission of Higher Education (WICHE) program and welcomes WICHE-sponsored students from Arizona, Hawaii, Montana, Nevada, New Mexico, North Dakota, and Wyoming.

> The Washington-Idaho-Montana-Utah (WIMU) Regional Program in veterinary medicine is a partnership.

*Washington State University*
Washington State University is in Pullman, a town in southeastern Washington. Located in the Palouse region of the Inland Northwest, Pullman offers the benefits of small-town living with the cultural richness of bigger city life. The 60,000 people who live in the communities of Pullman and neighboring town, Moscow, Idaho, enjoy a lifestyle that combines a beautiful country setting with the benefits of two major universities (University of Idaho is just a few miles away). WSU is also a member of the PAC-12 athletic conference, offering exciting sporting events throughout the year. With a true four-season climate, beautiful rivers, nearby mountains and scenic mountain lakes, it's easy to take advantage of a variety of excellent recreational activities including hiking, mountain biking, skiing, snowboarding, fishing, camping and white-water rafting.

The WSU College of Veterinary Medicine was founded in 1899 and is one of the longest established colleges of veterinary medicine in the country. Several major buildings house the Departments of Veterinary Clinical Sciences, Integrative Physiology and Neurosciences, Veterinary Microbiology and Pathology, and the School of Molecular Biosciences. The college also includes the Veterinary Teaching Hospital, the Washington Animal Disease Diagnostic Laboratory and the Paul G. Allen School for Global Animal Health.

Hands-on experience at WSU begins on day one with caseloads that provide extensive experience in all areas of interest including small animal, food animal, equine, and exotics. Because WSU clinicians have a wide-range of specialty areas, the Veterinary Teaching Hospital sees a large and diverse caseload. Students are encouraged to spend time in the Veterinary Teaching Hospital throughout all four years of study. The DVM program also allows for students to take advantage of numerous off-campus clinical opportunities in all areas of veterinary medicine. There are interactive case opportunities at our satellite clinics in Spokane, WA and Caldwell, ID, and our affiliate preceptor clinics scattered throughout the northwest.

The WSU College of Veterinary Medicine is also a leader of innovative educational programs. Before students even take their first veterinary class, they begin their education with the Cougar Orientation and Leadership Experience (COLE), an on-site and off-site retreat designed to promote collaboration and team building. By the time students enter their second year, they have already studied ethics, service, and leadership in veterinary medicine. In their second and

**PREREQUISITES FOR ADMISSION**

**Course requirements and semester hours**

| | |
|---|---|
| Biology (with lab) | 8 |
| Inorganic chemistry (with lab) | 8 |
| Organic chemistry (with lab) | 4 |
| Physics (with lab) | 4 |
| Math (algebra or higher) | 3 |
| Genetics | 3-4 |
| Biochemistry | 3 |
| Statistical methods | 3 |
| Arts/Humanities/Social Sciences/History* | 21 |
| English composition/Communication* | 6 |
| **TOTAL** | **64** |

*General education requirements will be waived if a student has a bachelor's degree.

third years, students take classes to learn skills in clinical communication, diagnostic reasoning and may elect to take courses on how to manage a veterinary practice as a part of the Veterinary Business Management Association Certificate Program. The Paul G. Allen School for Global Animal Health builds on the college's rich history of research on animal diseases that directly impact human health and offers DVM students the opportunity to earn a Professional Certificate in Global Animal Health. The program is coordinated through the Allen School in partnership with other departments and schools at WSU and the University of Washington's Department of Global Health (School of Medicine and School of Public Health).

*Utah State University*
Utah State University is nationally and internationally recognized for its research in animal and biomedical sciences. USU's School of Veterinary Medicine offers an affordable, academically outstanding path to pursue a professional degree in veterinary medicine. Classes are taught by faculty from the Department of Animal, Dairy, and Veterinary Sciences and are held in state-of-the-art teaching facilities on the Logan, Utah campus. With dedicated faculty and only 30 students per class, students will experience a supportive environment for active learning. Students spend their first two years in Logan and then transfer to Pullman for their remaining two years.

Cache Valley is one of Utah's hidden treasures, and Logan, with its population of just under 50,000 residents, sits at the heart of it. Cache Valley lies 83 miles north of Salt Lake City and is a land of dairy farms, small towns, and friendly people. The majestic mountains provide outstanding all-season outdoor recreation, and there are plenty of historical, musical, and art events, plus numerous dining, lodging, and shopping offerings.

*Montana State University*
Montana State University is a public university located in Bozeman, Montana. It is the state's land grant university and primary campus in the Montana State University System. MSU is ranked in the top tier of US research institutions by the Carnegie Foundation for the Advancement of Teaching. Classes will be taught by faculty from several departments, including those individuals that already participate in the instruction of medical students in the human medical WWAMI program. The Montana residents will spend their first year in Bozeman and then transfer to Pullman for their remaining three years.

Bozeman is located in the beautiful Gallatin Valley, and is a safe and supportive community offering significant opportunity to combine a fantastic educational experience with the great outdoors. Bozeman has a population close to 40,000 residents, making it the fourth largest city in Montana. The area offers fantastic hiking and backpacking opportunities in the surrounding mountain ranges, and the skiing and fishing is some of the best in the country. Yellowstone National Park is a short drive to the south, offering year round recreational activities.

*WIMU and WICHE Program Details*

Students applying as Washington residents are competing for up to 55 spots for Washington residents only. Students applying as Idaho residents are competing for up to 11 spots for Idaho residents only. Students accepted from the Washington and Idaho pools will complete all four years on the WSU Pullman campus. The joint program between WSU/USU will seat up to 20 Utah residents and up to 10 non-resident, non-sponsored students to spend their first two years in Logan, Utah. Much of the curriculum will be taught by the faculty of USU's Department of Animal, Dairy, and Veterinary Sciences, paralleling the curriculum taught in Pullman. The final two years are completed at the WSU Pullman campus. Students applying as Montana residents are competing for 10 spots for Montana residents only as a part of the regional cooperative program. Students selected for this joint program will spend their first year in Bozeman, Montana, where classes—which parallel those in Pullman—are taught by experienced health science educators who have instructed medical students in the University of Washington's WWAMI Medical Education Program. The final three years are completed at the WSU Pullman campus. There are up to 25 spots available for WICHE-sponsored and non-resident, non-sponsored students at the WSU Pullman Campus.

Upon satisfactory completion of our program, the Doctor of Veterinary Medicine (DVM) degree is conferred by the Regents of Washington State University. Although the University of Idaho, Montana State University, and Utah State University are partners in the program, all students receive their DVM degrees from WSU.

## APPLICATION INFORMATION

All applicants, regardless of residency, must complete the VMCAS application and WIMU/WSU Supplemental Application. Applicants must declare their state of residency on the VMCAS and WIMU/WSU Supplemental Application. By identifying yourself as a Washington resident, Idaho resident, Montana resident, Utah resident, a resident of a WICHE state (Arizona, Hawaii, Montana, Nevada, New Mexico, North Dakota, Wyoming), or as a non-sponsored, non-resident, your application will be funneled through the appropriate application pool. It is highly recommended that applicants contact the appropriate state authority for information regarding residency requirements as early in the application process as possible.

For the most current application information (availability, deadlines, fees, and VMCAS participation), please refer to www.vetmed.wsu.edu/ProspectiveStudents as well as the contact information listed above.

Residency implications: In general, first preference is given to qualified applicants who are residents of Washington, Idaho, Montana, Utah, and qualified applicants sponsored by WICHE contract states. Second preference is given to qualified non-resident, non-sponsored applicants.

At the Pullman site there are up to 55 available seats for Washington residents, up to 11 for Idaho residents, and up to 25 for WICHE-sponsored and non-resident, non-sponsored students.

At the Logan site there are up to 20 available seats for Utah residents and up to 10 for non-resident, non-sponsored students.

At the Montana site there are up to 10 available seats for Montana residents.

## SUMMARY OF ADMISSIONS PROCEDURES

*Timetable*

*VMCAS application deadline:* Thursday, October 2, 2014 1:00 PM Eastern Time

*WIMU/WSU Supplemental deadline:* Thursday, October 9, 2014 by 5 PM Pacific Time (The supplemental application can be accessed at: www.vetmed.wsu.edu/ProspectiveStudents)

*Interview dates:* November-February

*Acceptance letters mailed:* November-April

*School begins:* late August

*Deposit (to hold place in class):* none required

*Deferments:* considered on a case-by-case basis

## EVALUATION CRITERIA

Applicants are selected based upon ability to successfully complete the program and demonstration of the qualities that make a successful veterinarian. Academic criteria include grades, quality and rigor of academic program and GRE test scores. Non-academic factors include animal, veterinary, research, and work experience; honors and awards; community service and extracurricular activities; written essay; and letters of recommendation. Other factors include maturity, integrity, compassion, communication skills, and desire to contribute to society. An interview is required for Washington, Idaho, Montana and Utah residents, as well as for non-resident, non-sponsored applicants. WICHE applicants who are certified as residents of their contract state are ranked for participation in the WICHE program using the same criteria above minus the interview.

## 2013 ADMISSIONS SUMMARY

| | Number of Applicants | Number of New Entrants |
|---|---|---|
| Washington | 155 | 57 |
| Idaho | 37 | 11 |
| Utah | 51 | 18 |
| WICHE states | 204 | 28 |
| (9 WICHE sponsored) | | |
| Nonresident | 722 | 19 |
| **Total** | **1,169** | **133** |
| (101 Pullman / 32 Logan) | | |

## EXPENSES FOR THE 2013-2014 ACADEMIC YEAR

*Tuition and fees - Pullman Site*

*Resident (WA, ID, and WICHE supported):* $22,352

*Nonresident:* $53,406

*Tuition and fees - Bozeman Site*

*Resident:* $23,345

*Tuition - Logan Site*

*Resident:* $21,830

*Nonresident with scholarship:* $44,884

*Nonresident without scholarship:* $52,884

## ENTRANCE REQUIREMENTS

*Required undergraduate GPA:* No minimum requirement. A minimum overall GPA of 3.20 on a 4.00 scale is recommended.

*AP credit policy:* Must meet Washington State University requirements.

*Course completion deadline:* Prerequisite courses must be completed before time of matriculation.

*Standardized examinations:* Graduate Record Examination (GRE) General Test is required. Test scores older than 5 years will not be accepted. Test scores are due by October 2, 2014.

## ADDITIONAL REQUIREMENTS AND CONSIDERATIONS

Animal/veterinary/research/work experience

Letters of Recommendation. Both an academic and DVM letter are required. A minimum of three letters and a maximum of six letters will be reviewed by the admissions committee.

Extracurricular and community service activities, honors and awards

Personal Statement

WIMU/WSU Supplemental Application

*Is a Bachelor's Degree Required?* no

*Is this an International School?* no

## TEST REQUIREMENTS

*Standardized examinations:* Graduate Record Examination (GRE) General Test is required. Test scores older than 5 years will not be accepted. Test scores are due by October 2, 2014.

*VMCAS Participation:* full

*Accepts International Students?* yes

## ADDITIONAL INFORMATION

*VMCAS Application Deadline:* 10/2/2014

*WIMU/WSU Application Deadline:* 10/9/2014

# WESTERN UNIVERSITY OF HEALTH SCIENCES

Email Address: admissions@westernu.edu

Website: http://www.prospective.westernu.edu/veterinary/requirements

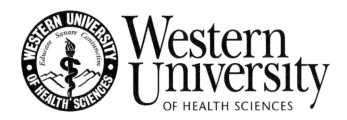

## SCHOOL DESCRIPTION

Western University of Health Sciences is an independent, accredited, nonprofit university incorporated in the State of California, dedicated to educating compassionate and competent health professionals who value diversity and a humanistic approach to patient care. The university, located in the San Gabriel Valley of Southern California, about 30 miles east of Los Angeles, grants post baccalaureate professional degrees in nine colleges: the College of Podiatric Medicine, the College of Dental Medicine, the College of Optometry, the Graduate College of Biomedical Sciences, the College of Allied Health Professions, the College of Graduate Nursing, the College of Osteopathic Medicine of the Pacific, the College of Pharmacy, and the College of Veterinary Medicine. The American Veterinary Medical Association Council on Education granted the College of Veterinary Medicine full accreditation status in 2010. Western U's CVM admitted its charter class Fall 2003. The founding principles of the College of Veterinary Medicine include:

> Western University is dedicated to educating compassionate and competent health professionals.

1. Commitment to student-centered, life-long learning. The curriculum is designed to teach students to find and critically evaluate information, to enhance student cooperative learning, and to provide an environment for professional development.

2. Commitment to a Reverence for Life philosophy in teaching veterinary medicine. The College strives to make the educational experience one that enhances moral development of its students and is respectful to all animals and people involved in its programs. Students only practice clinical and surgical skills on live animals when it is medically necessary for that animal.

3. Commitment to excellence of student education through strategic partnerships in the public and private veterinary sectors.

This commitment seeks to maximize the learning experience in veterinary clinical practice and to educate practice-ready veterinarians capable of functioning independently upon graduation. In the 3rd and 4th years of the curriculum students are trained primarily off-campus at state of the art facilities.

## APPLICATION INFORMATION

For specific application information (availability, deadlines, fees, and VMCAS participation), please refer to the contact information listed previously.

*Residency implications:* applicants from all states as well as international applicants will be considered. In-state and out-of-state applicants are given equal consideration.

## SUMMARY OF ADMISSION PROCEDURES

*Timetable*

*VMCAS application deadline:* Thursday, October 2, 2014 1:00 PM Eastern Daylight Time

*Supplemental application deadline:* electronically submitted with the prerequisite worksheet received on or before October 2, 2014 at 12:00 PM PDT

## PREREQUISITES FOR ADMISSION

| Course Description | Number of Hours/Credits | Necessity |
| --- | --- | --- |
| Organic Chemistry with Lab | 3 | Required |
| Biochemistry or Physiological Chemistry | 3 | Required |
| Upper-Division Biological and Life Sciences with Lab | 9 | Required |
| Microbiology | 3 | Required |
| Upper-Division Physiology (Animal, Human, or Comparative Only) | 3 | Required |
| Genetics | 3 | Required |
| General or College Physics with Labs | 6 | Required |
| Statistics (General, Introductory, or Bio-) | 3 | Required |
| English Composition | 6 | Required |
| Humanities/Social Sciences | 9 | Required |

*Date interviews are held:* November-December

*Date acceptances mailed:* January

*School begins:* August

*Deposit (to hold place in class):* $500

*Deferments:* request for deferments will be considered on a case-by-case basis and only after deposit is received.

## EVALUATION CRITERIA

Academic achievement

Standardized test performance

Animal experience

Letters of reference

Interview

Other supporting material

Entrance Requirements

*Required undergraduate GPA:* Applicants must have a minimum overall GPA of 2.75 (undergraduate and graduate) at the time of application to be considered for admission. Prerequisite courses must be completed with a grade of C (or its equivalent) or higher. GPA must be maintained through matriculation into the program.

*AP credit policy:* must appear on official college transcripts and be equivalent to the appropriate college-level coursework. AP test subject and number of credits must also be specified on the transcript.

*Is a Bachelor's Degree Required?* no

*Is this an International School?* no

## ESTIMATED TUITION

*Estimated Tuition Resident:* $49,595.00

*Estimated Tuition Contract:* $0

*Estimated Tuition Non-Resident:* $49,595.00

## AVAILABLE SEATS

*Resident:* 47

*Contract:* 0

*Non-Resident:* 53

## TEST REQUIREMENTS

*Standardized examinations:* Graduate Record Examination (GRE), general test, or Medical College Admissions Test (MCAT) is required. Test scores must be received by the Admissions Office on or before October 2, 2014.

*VMCAS Participation:* full

*Accepts International Students?* yes

## ADDITIONAL INFORMATION

All courses must be completed at a regionally accredited college or university in the United States. Exceptions will be made on a case-by-case basis.

Coursework completed outside the U.S. (including Canada) must be evaluated by a WesternU approved evaluation service (please visit the requirements page of the website for a listing of approved services).

All required courses must be completed by the end of the spring term of planned matriculation year.

Failure to satisfactorily complete prerequisites with a grade of C or better will result in the loss of a candidate's seat in the class.

One course cannot be used to satisfy more than one prerequisite.

While not specifically required, courses in anatomy, nutrition, immunology, and embryology are strongly encouraged.

All except two of the science prerequisite courses must be completed by the end of the Fall term immediately prior to the planned year of matriculation at WesternU-CVM.

*Application Deadline:* 10/2/2014

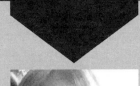
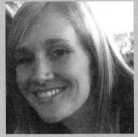

**What has been your favorite thing about attending veterinary school so far?**
My favorite thing is interacting with the clients and patients I see at the hospital. I know there are people and animals that I have effected positively. My work has made a difference in their lives. It is an amazing feeling. Seeing the animal and owners reunite after a troubling experience—and seeing both of them so happy—is something truly special.

**What advice do you have for prospective veterinary school applicants?**
Think long and hard before applying to veterinary school. Veterinary school is stressful and takes an almost unimaginable amount of work and dedication. In order to succeed, your education must be a priority. Social life is secondary. That being said, if you are determined to become a veterinarian, and have the required devotion to reach your goal, then give it your best effort and stay focused. Keep in mind, there are a lot of people who would like to be in your shoes.

**What are your short-term and long-term goals?**
My short-term career goal at this moment is to find a job at a small animal general practice with a great mentor. I know I have much more to learn and hope to find someone who supports me in my educational progress. I would love to obtain a certification in physical therapy. I have also found that I am particularly interested in neurology and surgery. Although internships are not in the future for me, I would like to broaden my knowledge base in those fields as much as possible. My long-term career goals are still being established. I know that I want to be successful and continue learning and staying up-to-date with the medical field. I hope to be a partner at a practice one day as well.

**What was the biggest challenge you faced during veterinary school?**
My biggest challenge was balancing school and being a single mother. Trying to figure out my schedule and babysitter availability, along with keeping all of my schoolwork up-to-date, left little time to relax. I'm very proud of myself for accomplishing what I have. Anything is possible if you want it badly enough.

**Do you plan to practice veterinary medicine after graduating from veterinary school?**
Yes, this has been my dream since I was five years old. I can't believe it is almost accomplished! I love every aspect of the career—the medicine, the animals, and the clients. There is not another profession that allows you to practice so many different aspects of medicine, such as surgery, neurology, internal medicine, emergency, radiology, cardiology, ophthalmology, and so forth. I can't wait to see what I really know once I start practicing.

**What advice do you have for other students who are currently in veterinary school?**
The advice I have for other students who are currently in veterinary school is to "just keep swimming." I know the end seems so far away, but it will fly by. Cherish the time you have here, and realize that you are here to learn. It is okay to tell a clinician when you don't know something. It is okay to ask questions. Take advantage of the opportunity to gain greater experience and knowledge whenever possible. You may not get the chance to ask that question when you are out in practice. Realize that even though you may feel like an idiot some days, you're not. Just keep doing the best you can.

**Why do you want to be a veterinarian?**
I have always loved animals, but I have also loved being around people. I noticed the impact veterinarians had on human's lives as well as the animal world when I started working in the veterinary field at the age of sixteen. I also love puzzles, and medicine is like a puzzle to me. Basically, I want to be a veterinarian because I know I will wake up every morning excited to get on with my day. I won't be working, because I will love what I do.

# UNIVERSITY OF WISCONSIN

Email Address: oaa@vetmed.wisc.edu
Website: http://www.vetmed.wisc.edu

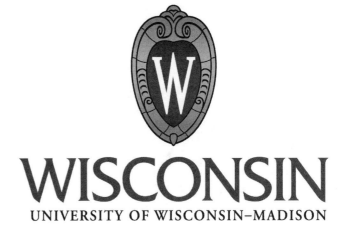

## SCHOOL DESCRIPTION

The University of Wisconsin is located in Madison, the state capital, which has a population of about 230,000. Consistently ranked among the nation's "most livable" cities, its hilly terrain, scattered parks, and woodlands saturate the urban setting with a friendly neighborhood atmosphere. Centered on a narrow isthmus among 4 scenic lakes, the city is a recreational paradise. The university sprawls over 900 acres along Lake Mendota and its student population is nearly 45,000. It has rated among the top 10 universities academically since 1910 and is third in the country in volume of research activity.

> The University of Wisconsin rated among the top 10 universities academically since 1910.

The School of Veterinary Medicine facility has a modern veterinary medical teaching hospital, modern equipment, and high-quality lab space for teaching and research. The curriculum provides a broad education in veterinary medicine with learning experiences in food animal medicine and other specialty areas. The school pioneered a unique senior rotation in ambulatory service for fourth-year students where they experience the life and work of a veterinarian specializing in large-animal medicine by completing a rotation in one of 22 practices near Madison. The school has an outstanding research program and many faculty members have joint appointments with the College of Agricultural and Life Sciences, the School of Medicine and Public Health, the Regional Primate Center, the McArdle Cancer Research Institute, the National Wildlife Health Laboratory, and the North Central Dairy Forage Center. These outside links provide learning, research, and employment opportunities for students.

## APPLICATION INFORMATION

To apply for admission, all applicants must complete three (3) online applications: 1) VMCAS, due October 2, 2014 (1:00 PM, EDT); 2) Wisconsin's Required Data Form, due October 2, 2014 (1:00 PM, CDT) and located at our website: www.vetmed.wisc.edu/dvm-students/prospective-students/ ; and 3) Wisconsin's Supplemental Application. All applicants will be notified by e-mail in November 2014 to complete our electronic supplemental application and to announce its deadline. Interviews are not required as part of the application process.

For specific application information (availability, deadlines, fees, and VMCAS participation), please refer to the contact information listed above.

*Residency implications:* between 60 and 70 Wisconsin residents will be accepted. Wisconsin has no contractual agreements, but may accept 17-27 nonresidents. Applicants who can claim legal residency or domicile in more than one state should contact the school.

## SUMMARY OF ADMISSION PROCEDURES

*Timetable*

*VMCAS application deadline:* Thursday, October 2, 2014 1:00 PM Eastern Time

*Interviews:* none

*Date acceptances mailed:* late-February

*School begins:* late August

*Deposit (to hold place in class):* none required.

## PREREQUISITES FOR ADMISSION

| Course Description | Number of Hours/Credits | Necessity |
|---|---|---|
| Biology or Zoology | 4 | Required |
| Genetics or Animal Breeding | 3 | Required |
| General Chemistry | 8 | Required |
| Organic Chemistry | 3 | Required |
| Biochemistry | 3 | Required |
| General Physics | 6 | Required |
| Statistics | 3 | Required |
| English Composition or Journalism | 6 | Required |
| Social Science or Humanities | 6 | Required |
| Anatomy | 3 | Recommended |
| Microbiology | 3 | Recommended |
| Physiology | 3 | Recommended |
| Cell/Molecular Biology | 3 | Recommended |

*Deferments:* are considered on an individual basis by the Admissions Committee and may be granted for extenuating circumstances.

## EVALUATION CRITERIA

There is a 2-part admission procedure. For the fall 2013 application year, the class was selected based upon the following comparative evaluation:

1. Evaluation of academic record
   Undergraduate cumulative GPA
   Required course GPA
   Most recent 30 semester credit GPA
   GRE test scores

2. Evaluation of personal experience and characteristics
   Animal and veterinary work experience
   Other preparatory experience (includes extracurricular activities)
   Personal history/academic performance (summary category to include review of academic history, academic achievements, diversity of background, etc.)
   Letters of recommendation

## ENTRANCE REQUIREMENTS

*Required undergraduate GPA:* A minimum grade of C (2.0) must be earned in all required courses, including courses completed after application. The mean undergraduate cumulative GPA for the class of 2017 was 3.65 for residents and 3.70 for nonresidents.

*AP credit policy:* must appear on official college transcripts and be equivalent to the appropriate college-level coursework.

*Is a Bachelor's Degree Required?* no

*Is this an International School?* no

## ESTIMATED TUITION

Tuition rates are published each year in July; please see our website for details.

*2013-2014 Estimated Tuition Resident:* $19,055.04

*Estimated Tuition Contract:* n/a

*2013-2014 Estimated Tuition Non-Resident:* $25,899.36

## TEST REQUIREMENTS

Standardized examinations: Graduate Record Examination (GRE), general test, is required. All applicants are required to take or retake the GRE, including the writing assessment. The GRE may be taken no later than October 1, 2014.

A test of English as a foreign language (TOEFL, MELAB, or IELTS scores may be submitted) is required for applicants for whom English is a second language and have not completed an undergraduate degree at an English-speaking college or university. The minimum scores accepted are as follows: internet TOEFL = 100, computer TOEFL = 250, paper TOEFL = 600, MELAB - 84, IELTS = 7. This must be taken no later than October 1, 2014. Please see website for additional information.

*VMCAS Participation:* full

*Accepts International Students?* yes

*Application Deadline:* 10/02/2014

# INTERNATIONAL
## VETERINARY MEDICAL SCHOOLS
*AVMA/COE Accredited*

# UNIVERSITY OF CALGARY

University of Calgary Faculty of Veterinary Medicine
Email Address: vet.admissions@ucalgary.ca
Website: http://vet.admissions@ucalgary.ca

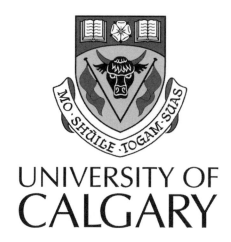

UNIVERSITY OF
# CALGARY

## SCHOOL DESCRIPTION

The University of Calgary Faculty of Veterinary Medicine (UCVM) offers a four-year professional degree leading to a Doctor of Veterinary Medicine (DVM). Completion of at least 4 or more semesters of full-time post-secondary instruction at a recognized university or at a college providing university-equivalency in coursework is required prior to application to the DVM program.

> The University of Calgary Faculty of Veterinary Medicine (UCVM) offers a four-year professional degree leading to a DVM.

## APPLICATION INFORMATION

Application Information Application forms for the Faculty of Veterinary Medicine are available on the website (vet. ucalgary.ca/dvmprogram). Applications will be considered from those students meeting the residency, English and academic admission requirements. Applications are to be submitted to the UCVM Office of Admissions by January 10. Two sets of official transcripts are required, one sent in by February 7 and the second should be sent as soon as final marks are available in the spring and no later than June 7. Transcripts should be sent directly to the UCVM Admissions Office.

Completed application forms include the following: complete personal information; a signed statement verifying Alberta residency status and verifying completion of the academic requirements; three letters of reference (required by January 10 with the application); post-secondary transcripts submitted by the appropriate aca-demic institution; a statement of work experience; and a statement of major extra-curricular activities.

English language proficiency must be demonstrated for all applicants for whom English is not their first language. English language proficiency can be demonstrated in one of the following ways:

(a) Completion of at least two full years within a degree program offered by an accredited university in a country which the University of Calgary recognizes as English language proficiency exempt.

(b) A minimum score of 92 on the internet based TOEFL (Test of English as a Foreign Language) and a minimum score of 50 on the Test of Spoken English (TSE); or a minimum score of 237 on the computer based TOEFL and a minimum score of 50 on the TSE; or a minimum score of 580 on the paper based TOEFL and a minimum score of 50 on the TSE.

## SUMMARY OF ADMISSIONS PROCEDURES

Enrolment in the DVM program at UCVM is currently limited to approximately 32 students who are Alberta residents. The Admissions Committee selects students for the program on the basis of academic and non-academic factors. Students are assessed academically on performance in their last 4 full undergraduate semesters and in the required courses. Applicants meeting the academic eligibility requirements are invited for an interview day where non-academic factors are assessed. At interview day, applicants are required to complete an on-site essay and participate in a series of interviews and other activities. Applicants must attend interview day at their own expense. There is no entrance exam or requirement to complete the MCAT or GRE exams.

The admissions process identifies applicants who will flourish in a DVM program that prepares students for all aspects of veterinary medicine. Consistent with the UCVM mandate, preference will be given to applicants who demonstrate an interest in pursuing careers in general veterinary practice that support rural development and sustainability, and careers in the areas of emphasis. There is no specific animal or veterinary-related experience required; however, demonstration and understanding of the veterinary profession and animal industries relevant to the applicant's career interests is expected.

Applicants will be notified of the Admissions Committee's decision in June.

## ENTRANCE REQUIREMENTS

All successful applicants are required to forward $200.00 deposit within 15 working days of notification of admission. Failure to do so may result in the position being assigned to another applicant. Such deposits will be applied to the first year's fees. An applicant who accepts a position but later rescinds his or her acceptance will forfeit the entire $200.00 deposit. Successful applicants are required to have or receive immunization for tetanus and rabies following admission.

*Is a Bachelor's Degree Required?* no

*Is this an International School?* no

## ESTIMATED TUITION

*Estimated Tuition Resident:* $11,000.00

*Estimated Tuition Contract:* $0

*Estimated Tuition Non-Resident:* $0

*VMCAS Participation:* no

*Accepts International Students?* no

## ADDITIONAL INFORMATION

*Application Deadline:* January 10

# CENTRAL LUZON STATE UNIVERSITY

Office of the Dean
Science City of Muñoz 3120
Philippines
Phone: +63 44 4565877
Email Address: clsu@clsu.edu.ph
Website: http://clsucvsm.edu.ph/

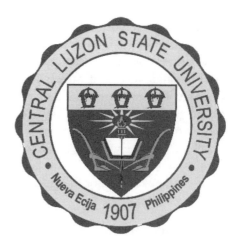

## SCHOOL DESCRIPTION

Central Luzon State University (CLSU) is located on a 658-hectare sprawling main campus in the Science City of Muñoz, which is located 150 kilometers north of Manila. It also has a more than 1000-hectare site for ranch type buffalo production and forestry development up the hills of Carranglan town, in northern Nueva Ecija, 40 kilometers away from the main campus. The University is the lead agency of the Muñoz Science Community and the seat of the Regional Research and Development Center in Central Luzon. To date, CLSU is one of the premier institutions of agriculture in Southeast Asia known for its breakthrough researches in aquaculture (pioneer in the sex reversal of Tilapia), ruminants, crops, orchard, and water management researches.

> For many years, DVM graduates from CVSM have consistently topped the Veterinary Licensure Examinations in the country.

The College of Veterinary Science and Medicine (CVSM) was established in 1978 through Republic Act No. 4067 enacted into law by Congress in 1964. Subsequently, CVSM offered the first ladderized veterinary curriculum in the Philippines: Bachelor of Science in Animal Husbandry (first 4 years) and Doctor of Veterinary Medicine (6 years). This was designed to produce veterinarians adept not only in disease control and prevention but in animal production as well. For many years, DVM graduates from CVSM have consistently topped the Veterinary Licensure Examinations in the country. This excellent performance has made the Philippine Commission on Higher Education (CHED) and the Professional Regulation Commission (PRC) to recognize the CVSM as one of the Top Performing Veterinary Colleges in the country. In 2009, CHED awarded the college the title, Center of Excellence in Veterinary Medicine.

## APPLICATION INFORMATION

The following are the admission requirements for both undergraduate and graduate programs:

## UNDERGRADUATE PROGRAM

1. Grade Point Average of 2.25 or better in the first year
2. Passing the interview and qualifying examination conducted by the college admission committee
3. Submission of duly accomplished application form and four copies of two 2" x 2" photos
4. Passing the National Veterinary Admission Test for the DVM program

*For Transferees*

1. Certificate of Honorable Dismissal and Transcript of Records
2. Certificate of Good Moral Character issued by the dean or director of student services of the school last attended
3. Compliance with the general admission requirements of the university and those of the college

*For Foreign Students*

1. Presentation and submission of authenticated passport and visa
2. Alien Certificate of Registration
3. Study Permit

4. Transcript of Records
5. Certificate of Eligibility for Admission issued by the Commission on Higher Education
6. Compliance with the general admission requirements of the university
7. All other government requirements
8. Students from countries where English is not a medium of instruction must pass the English proficiency test administered by the Department of English and Humanities

## GRADUATE PROGRAM

A DVM degree or its equivalent from a recognized institution is a requirement along with the submission of the following:

1. Duly accomplished application form
2. Original or authenticated transcript of records showing a grade point average (GPA) of at least 2.0 or its equivalent.
3. Applicants with GPA below 2.0 may be admitted on a probationary status if recommended by the department chair and approved by the dean after thorough review of the applicant's qualification to do graduate work.
4. Two letters of recommendation from former professors in the undergraduate course.

*Is a Bachelor's Degree Required?* no

*Is this an International School?* yes

## ESTIMATED TUITION

*Estimated Tuition Resident:* Php 7,000.00 per semester

*Estimated Tuition Non-Resident (International):* Php 12,000.00 per semester

## AVAILABLE SEATS

*Resident:* N/A

*Non-Resident (International):* n/a

*VMCAS Participation:* non-VMCAS

*Accepts International Students?* yes

*Application Deadline:* Last week of April every year.

# UNIVERSITY COLLEGE DUBLIN

Veterinary Medicine Degree programme
VMCAS Veterinary Medicine Applications UCD Admissions Office
Tierney Building University College Dublin Belfield, Dublin 4
Ireland
Tel: 00 353 1 716 1555
Email: onlineapps@ucd.ie http://www.ucd.ie/vetmed/

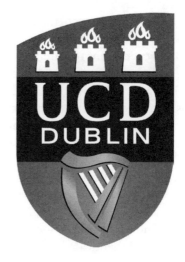

## SCHOOL DESCRIPTION

UCD is the sole provider of a veterinary medicine degree programme on the island of Ireland, and enjoys a long and proud tradition in the provision of veterinary education. Students of the veterinary medicine programme benefit from the outstanding facilities of the purpose-designed UCD Veterinary Sciences Centre and UCD Veterinary Hospital on the main university campus at Belfield, Dublin (commissioned in 2002). Located on a 132 Ha site 5km south of Dublin's City Centre, UCD is Ireland's largest university with over 23,000 students. This is complemented by Lyons Estate Farm where students have practical classes at all stages of the curriculum.

> The programme is designed to educate you to the best international standards in veterinary medicine.

As the gateway to Europe, Ireland has been renowned for learning and creativity for centuries. Our English-speaking, well-educated population has drawn global companies like Google, Facebook, Intel and HP, who now collaborate with us and employ our graduates.

With its unique blend of urban chic, lush parkland, sweeping coastline, fabulous shopping and excellent cultural experiences, Dublin is without a doubt one of the most energised capital cities in Europe.

Dublin at a Glance
- 8th best student city in the world
- Official UNESCO City of Literature
- European City of Science 2012
- Popular Dublin Bikes public cycling scheme
- Famous for music, literature and theatre
- 5000 acres of green space, including Europe's largest urban park
- Travel hub for easy access to Europe
- EU headquarters for Google, Facebook and many other international MNCs

UCD is a diverse, International campus. Our student population comprises of more than 50 nationalities, and international students now account for one-third of the total undergraduate student cohort. This diversity is one of the defining features of life at UCD, and one that enriches the student experience by delivering of a truly international campus. Your experience as a vet student will guarantee life-long friendships.

### Programme/Syllabus

Our veterinary programme is accredited by the Veterinary Council of Ireland, the American Veterinary Medical Association, and the European Association of Establishments in Veterinary Education. Our programme is designed to educate you to the best international standards in veterinary medicine and to prepare you for entry to any branch of the veterinary profession. Veterinary medicine is concerned with the promotion of the health and welfare of animals of special importance to society. This involves the care of healthy and sick animals, the prevention, recognition, control and treatment of their diseases and the welfare and productivity of livestock. Veterinarians also safeguard human health through prevention and control of diseases transmitted from animals to man, through ensuring the safety of foods of animal origin, and through advancing the science and art of comparative medicine.

Veterinary graduates have a wide spectrum of careers to choose from including private practice (companion animals, food animals, horses, exotics, or a mixture of these), in government service (animal health, food safety, public health), in research or in industry.

US applicants through VMCAS are eligible to apply to enter this programme provided they have the prerequisites as outlined below. Further curricular details are published on our web site, www.ucd.ie/vetmed.

The Programme is organised into four stages. During Stage 2 students will take combined modules with students on the Veterinary Medicine programme aimed at school-leavers. In Semesters 1 and 2 of the programme students will build on their knowledge of the basic biological sciences by taking modules designed to demonstrate how this knowledge is applied in the practice of veterinary medicine, and gain a firm grounding in animal welfare, behaviour and handling. A key objective will be to ensure that students have the required knowledge, skills and competences to progress to Stage 2. As the programme progresses students will learn clinical skills and study each of the clinical sciences using a "body systems" approach. Beginning in stage 1 students are required to complete a minimum of 34 weeks of practical extra-mural experience to be completed by stage 4 according to the specifications/ regulations for Extra Mural Studies (EMS). The final year of the programme consists of clinical rotations in UCD where students have the opportunity to work alongside experienced and specialist staff clinicians, and participate in patient care and client communication. Each student has a personalized timetable ensuring that they participate in rotations in Large and Small Animal Surgeries, Diagnostic Imaging, Anesthesiology, Small and Large Animal Medicine, Emergency Medicine, Clinical Reproduction, Herd Health, Population Medicine, Diagnostic Pathology, a rotation in shelter medicine is provided in collaboration with the Dogs Trust, and Clinical Pathology. Assessments at the end of this clinical year are through Objective Structured Clinical Examinations (OSCEs) and Clinical Proficiency Examinations (CPEs). Throughout the programme students are required to participate in extra-mural studies. In the early years, this consists of gaining experience in the handling and management of farm and companion animals, and in later years, of working with veterinarians in practice (clinical extra-mural experience).

## APPLICATION INFORMATION

For specific application information (availability, fees and VMCAS participation), please refer to the contact information listed above. For further information on entry to the Republic of Ireland, please refer to www.educationireland.com (i.e., students must also be able to ensure adequate financial support for the duration of their programme).

## SUMMARY OF ADMISSION PROCEDURE

*Timetable*

*VMCAS application deadline:* Thursday, October 2, 2014 at 1:00 PM Eastern Time

*Interviews:* January through to March (held in the US)

*Date Acceptances Mailed:* Early April

*Deposit (to hold place in class):* €2,000, required by early March

*Deferments:* Not applicable

## EVALUATION CRITERIA

Academic performance

References/evaluations (minimum 2 required-one from academic science source and one from a veterinary surgeon)

1 page personal statement Animal & Veterinary Experience

Interview

## 2012-2013 ADMISSIONS SUMMARY (FOR ENTRY IN 2013)

|  | Number of Applicants | Number of New Entrants |
|---|---|---|
| In-province | 909 | 90 |
| International | 221 | 37 |
| Total | 1,130 | 137 |

## EXPENSES FOR THE 2014-2015

*Annual tuition and fees*

*EU Graduate:* €19,500

*Non EU Graduate:* €33,500

## ADMISSION PROCESS

US and Canadian residents must apply to UCD through VMCAS and a supplemental application form which is available at www.ucd.ie/ vetmed.

Completed applications are reviewed by our admissions team. Successful applicants will receive their offers from January onwards. Classes begin in early September with compulsory orientation taking place prior to the start of classes.

**ENTRANCE REQUIREMENTS** Up to 30 places will be available in 2014 for overseas students. We look for a GPA of 3.2 or above.

All additional information required by UCD including the completed online supplemental application and supporting documentation by Saturday, 1st November 2014.

* For up-to-date information on fees and all further information regarding admission to the University College Dublin, please visit our web site www.ucd.ie.

# VETERINARIAN PROFILE: MEGAN NOYES

**YEAR OF GRADUATION**
2010

**PLACE OF EMPLOYMENT**
Glen Erin Animal Hospital

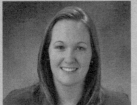

### What is your favorite aspect of being a veterinarian?
I really enjoy the problem-solving aspect of this career. There is a lot of repetition in this field and it can be monotonous at times. However, when you get to break out of the box and do something new it can be very exciting. Every now and then a case turns out differently than you expect or is atypical in some way, and you have to find new solutions to the problem. You have to stretch your skills and comfort zone, and that can be really fun and interesting. I also really love interacting with the animals. Every now and then you get a first kitten visit or a really happy dog and it can make everything else brighter. In the end, we really are doing all of it for the animals, and enjoying them is incredibly important.

### What type of veterinary medicine do you practice?
I spend most of my time working on preventive and internal medicine of dogs and cats. Occasionally, I also get to do internal medicine of rabbits and pocket pets.

### Where did you attend veterinary school?
I attended the Ontario Veterinary College in Guelph, Ontario, Canada.

### How long have you been practicing as a veterinarian?
I have been working full time as a veterinarian for four years.

### What advice do you have for those considering a career in veterinary medicine?
The best advice I can give is to gain as much hands-on experience as possible. There is so much more to this career than just loving animals or thinking that puppies and kittens are fun. It requires a lot of hard work, a huge emotional investment in each and every patient, and it requires that you can make tough decisions. The more time you spend in clinics or on farms, listening to veterinarians, listening to clients, and absorbing the experience of clinical practice, the more prepared you are to decide if veterinary medicine is the right path for you.

### What challenges have you faced while practicing veterinary medicine?
One of the biggest challenges in this field is the emotional investment required every day. We do this job because we care. It is not glamorous, it will not make you rich, and you do have to work nights, weekends, and holidays. We keep going to work every day because there is always just one more animal that we need to help. After a while it can become exhausting, giving your whole self to each and every patient and client. We call it compassion fatigue, and it is real. Facing that emotional exhaustion while continuing to provide good medicine for your patients is a big challenge. The second biggest challenge that we face is the cost of veterinary care. Our job would be infinitely easier if every pet had health insurance. We spend a significant part of our day explaining to clients why each test is important and why it is worth their money. Compared to our human counterparts, we have to make diagnoses and treatment plans based on a fraction of the diagnostic information that a medical doctor would have. This can become quite frustrating. It may also make us better doctors.

### What is your proudest moment of your veterinary career so far?
My proudest moments are always when I get hugs or thank-you notes from clients. Sometimes it is a hug because I have helped their pet, and sometimes it is a short note of gratitude because I was there when they said good-bye. It can absolutely surprise you, sometimes the people you think are the most unhappy with you turn out to be the people who are the most appreciative of you. The thanks let me know that I am doing my job well.

### What led you to pursue a career in veterinary medicine?
I came to veterinary medicine accidentally. All through high school I thought that I knew what I wanted to do with my life. After visiting several universities for marine biology, I realized that a lifetime of fish was not for me. I had a feeling that I wanted to work with animals in some way, but I had never considered veterinary medicine before. I began working at a small animal hospital in my senior year of high school purely because the opportunity came up. While I was working there I discovered that I really enjoyed the challenge of it, and I decided to apply to universities that held veterinary programs.

# UNIVERSITY OF EDINBURGH

Email Address: geraldine.giannopoulos@ed.ac.uk
Website: http://www.ed.ac.uk/schools-departments/vet

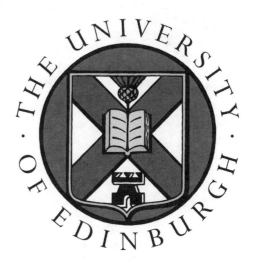

## SCHOOL DESCRIPTION

The Royal (Dick) School of Veterinary Studies, established in 1823, was the first veterinary school in Scotland, and the second to be established in the UK. The long-standing involvement of Edinburgh with veterinary education, where tradition is mixed with cutting-edge veterinary teaching, benefits from a closely-knit collegial community of "Dick" vet students. As one of only 15 international vet schools with AVMA accreditation, the veterinary degree course at Edinburgh (BVM&S) provides an excellent foundation for a subsequent career in veterinary practice or one of the many related career opportunities, such as biomedical research. The academic and research environment in Edinburgh is internationally recognized for encouraging excellence in a broad base of teaching and learning. The School is based at the Easter Bush one-site campus approximately 7 miles south of the city.

> Tradition is mixed with cutting-edge vet teaching and benefits from a closely-knit collegial community of vet students.

The city of Edinburgh, the capital of Scotland, is one of Europe's most handsome cities. The beauty of its setting and its architecture, allied with its intellectual traditions, have earned the title of "Athens of the North" for what is still a compact city of some 500,000 people. It is a city of noted buildings, fine gardens, and open spaces, including Holyrood Park—one of the largest city center natural parks in Europe—and Princes Street Gardens, between the Old and New Towns. The city offers students a rich mix of academic, social and allied facilities—libraries, museums and art galleries, concert halls, theaters and cinemas. The city has easy access to coastline, lochs, mountains and countryside, with ready-made opportunities for open-air sports and recreation. Further details on the BVM&S degree programme, the School and its facilities can be found by visiting http://www.ed.ac.uk/schools-departments/vet.

## APPLICATION INFORMATION

For specific application information (availability, deadlines, fees and VMCAS participation), please refer to the contact information listed above.

*Residency implications:* For full details and further information on entry to the UK, please refer to http://www.ukba.homeoffice.gov.uk. Please note that students must be able to ensure adequate financial support for the duration of their course. Candidates are not required to submit a supplemental application.

## SUMMARY OF ADMISSIONS PROCEDURES

*Timetable*

*VMCAS application deadline:* October 2, 2014 1:00 PM Eastern Time

*Receptions:* early to mid-February (held in the U.S.)

*Date acceptances mailed:* early April at the latest

*School begins:* mid-September or early August (for GEP entrants)

*Deposit (to hold place in class):* £1,500, required by early May

*Deferments:* Not applicable

## PREREQUISITES FOR ADMISSION

| Course Description | Number of Hours/Credits | Necessity |
|---|---|---|
| Physics | variable | Required |
| Biology/Zoology | variable | Required |
| Biochemistry | variable | Required |
| Organic Chemistry | variable | Required |
| Inorganic Chemistry | variable | Required |
| Mathematics/Statistics | variable | Required |
| Genetics | variable | Recommended |
| Microbiology | variable | Recommended |
| Cellular Biology | variable | Recommended |

## EVALUATION CRITERIA

Academic performance

GRE scores

Animal/veterinary experience

Personal statement

Motivation

References/Evaluations (minimum 2 required - one from academic science source and one from a veterinary surgeon)

## ENTRANCE REQUIREMENTS

*Graduate Entry (Undergraduate degree-holders or in senior year of degree)*

Candidates with a degree (or in their senior year) in an appropriate Biological or Animal Science degree may be considered for the 4-year BVM&S programme (Graduate Entry Programme). All applicants are required to have completed the required prerequisite courses for the programme. US applicants should have an overall minimum grade point average of 3.4 (4 point scale), with greater than 3.0 in science courses. The School also welcomes applications from candidates with an alternative degree who have also completed the required prerequisites. Candidates with a non-science degree would normally be considered for the 5-year BVM&S programme. However, if candidates have the specified prerequisites, they may be considered for the 4 year programme.

*Pre-Vet*

Candidates with two years of a pre-vet will be considered for the 5-year BVM&S programme. An overall GPA of 3.4 (4 point scale) is expected. All applicants are required to have completed the required prerequisite courses for the programme.

*Is a Bachelor's Degree Required?* no

*Is this an International School?* yes

## ESTIMATED TUITION

*Estimated Tuition Non-Resident:* £28,450

## AVAILABLE SEATS

*Resident:* 72

*Non-Resident:* 180

## TEST REQUIREMENTS

*Standardized examinations:* Graduate Record Examination (GRE) general test is required. The scores must be received by November 1 for 2015 entry. Applicants should ensure they take the GRE early enough for scores to be received before the deadline.

*VMCAS Participation:* partial

*Accepts International Students?* yes

## ADDITIONAL INFORMATION

Resident residents of the UK, who do not hold a first degree, are primarily government-funded International GBP £28,450 (fixed for duration of course) * For up-to-date information on fees and all further information regarding admission to the School, please visit our website www.ed.ac.uk/schools-departments/vet * further information on funding including estimated living costs for international students is available here: http://www.ed.ac.uk/schools-departments/student-funding/tuition-fees/undergraduate/tuition-fees.

*Application Deadline:* 10/2/2014 1:00 PM Eastern Time

# UNIVERSITY OF GLASGOW

Email Address: vet-sch-admissions@glasgow.ac.uk
Website: http://www.gla.ac.uk/schools/vet

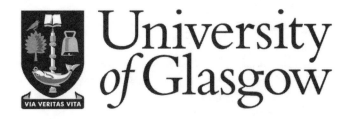

## SCHOOL DESCRIPTION

The School of Veterinary Medicine is located on the 80 hectare Garscube campus at the Northwest boundary of the city, four miles from the University's Gilmorehill campus. The School was founded in 1862 and gained independent Faculty status in 1969. In 2010, the Faculty translated from the "Faculty of Veterinary Medicine" to the "School of Veterinary Medicine" within the College of Medical, Veterinary and Life Sciences.

> The school is one of only five veterinary schools in Europe to be accredited to British, European and American standards.

The School has a 190 hectare commercial farm and research centre at Cochno, 15 minutes from the Garscube campus (5 miles north).

The city of Glasgow has a population of around 600,000 and is Scotland's largest city. One of Europe's liveliest places with a varied and colorful cultural and social life, it can cater to every taste. Situated on the River Clyde, Glasgow has excellent road and rail links to the rest of the UK and air services to a wide range of destinations, both home and overseas.

Wherever you come from, you can be sure of building friendships that last a lifetime at Glasgow. According to travel guide Lonely Planet, Glasgow is one of the world's top ten cities.

The School has approximately 199 staff (academic, research, and support) with an additional 65 postgraduate research students, 30 postgraduate clinical scholars, and 600 undergraduate students.

The school is pre-eminent in teaching, research, and clinical provision, and attracts students, researchers, and clinicians from around the world. Our internationally accredited school provides an expert referral centre via the Small Animal Hospital, the Weipers Centre for Equine Welfare, and the Scottish Centre for Production Animal Health & Welfare for animal owners and referring practitioners throughout the UK. In the Research Assessment Exercise 2008, the grade point average for our research activity was the highest in Scotland and joint highest in the UK, reaffirming our position as one of the country's leading veterinary schools.

Following the first ever international UK accreditation visit to be undertaken conjointly between the American Veterinary Medical Association (AVMA) Council on Education, the Royal College of Veterinary Surgeons (RCVS), the European Association of Establishments for Veterinary Education (EAEVE), and the Australasian Veterinary Boards Council (AVBC) in April 2013, the University of Glasgow's School of Veterinary Medicine has achieved full accreditation for a further period of seven years.

The BVMS programme is based on integration of clinical and science subject areas and has a spiral course structure, meaning that you will revisit topics as you progress through the programme, each time with increasing clinical focus. In conjunction, there is a vertical theme of professional and clinical skills development to help you acquire the personal qualities and skills you will need in professional environments.

The programme is delivered over five years and is divided into three phases. Years 1 and 2, Foundation Phase, Years 3 and 5, Clinical Phase, Year 5, Professional Phase.

## SPECIAL GLASGOW FEATURE

In common with all veterinary students in the UK, you will be required to undertake an additional 38 weeks of extra-mural studies (EMS) during your vacation time. The first period of 12 weeks is dedicated to gaining further experience of the management and handling of domestic animals. After this initial period is completed, you start the clinical period of 26 weeks, which can be used to gain experience in veterinary professional environments. Satisfactory completion of EMS is a requirement for graduation.

## APPLICATION INFORMATION

For specific application information (availability, deadlines, fees, and VMCAS participation), please refer to the contact information listed above.

*Residency implications:* Due to recent changes in immigration legislation, students from the U.S. (who are planning to come to the UK for more than 6 months) are now required to obtain an entry clearance certificate prior to entering the UK. For further information on entry to the UK, please refer to http://www.ukvisas.gov.uk . Students must also be able to ensure adequate financial support for the duration of their course.

## SUMMARY OF ADMISSIONS PROCEDURES

*Timetable*

*VMCAS application deadline:* Tuesday, October 2, 2014 1:00 PM Eastern Time

*Date interviews held:* January/February (In the US both East and West Coast)

*Date acceptances mailed:* April

*School begins:* late September

*Deposit (to hold place in class):* £1,000

*Deferments:* in certain circumstances

## EVALUATION CRITERIA

Academic performance
Animal/veterinary experience
References
Essay
Interview
Entrance Requirements
Course requirements
　Applicants are expected to have completed at least 2 years pre-veterinary or science courses at College or

University, with a minimum of one year in Chemistry (including organic chemistry and organic chemistry lab). We would expect high grades in all science subjects. US applicant should have a minimum 3.4 GPA (4 point scale), and to have achieved at 3.0 in Science.

*Required undergraduate GPA:* 3.40

*AP credit policy:* not applicable

*Course completion deadline:* required courses should be completed prior to admission in the fall.

*Standardized examinations:* none required. GRE results will be considered if submitted.

## ADDITIONAL REQUIREMENTS AND CONSIDERATIONS

Animal/veterinary work experience sufficient to indicate motivation, interest, and understanding of the veterinary profession
　Evaluations: minimum 2, one each from an academic science source and a veterinary surgeon.
　There is no supplemental application for the University of Glasgow.

*Is a Bachelor's Degree Required?* no

*Is this an International School?* yes

## ESTIMATED TUITION

*Resident of UK out with Scotland:* £9,000/yr

*International:* £25,000/yr (fixed at the point of entry)

## AVAILABLE SEATS

*Resident:* 72

*Non-Resident:* 55

## TEST REQUIREMENTS

*Standardized examinations:* none required. GRE results will be considered if submitted.

*VMCAS Participation:* partial

*Accepts International Students?* yes

## ADDITIONAL INFORMATION

For further information, contact the Undergraduate School Admissions Office (vet-sch-admissions@glasgow.ac.uk)

*Application Deadline:* 10/2/2014

# UNIVERSITY OF GUELPH

Email Address: vetmed@uoguelph.ca
Website: http://www.ovc.uoguelph.ca/recruitment/en/index.asp

**UNIVERSITY of GUELPH**

## SCHOOL DESCRIPTION

The Ontario Veterinary College (OVC) is a world leader in veterinary health care, learning and research.

We work at the intersection of animal, human, and ecosystem health.

Founded in 1862, OVC is the oldest veterinary school in Canada and the United States. OVC is located in Ontario, at the University of Guelph, and is a short drive from one of Canada's largest and well-known hubs of activity and culture, Toronto. A drive north takes you to the first of Canada's many popular lakes, known for clear waters and havens of nature.

> The Ontario Veterinary College works at the intersection of animal, human, and ecosystem health.

Academically, OVC is consistently ranked as one of Canada's top universities. In fact, we're renowned worldwide for excellence in teaching, research and service, with graduates of the program practicing veterinary medicine, conducting research or working in related industry across the globe.

With faculty and administration sharing like-minded ideas on furthering animal care, research and innovative teaching methodologies, OVC offers a rich and intense learning environment to students. Teaching hospital and facilities specialize in large and small animals , with dedicated intensive and oncology care, mean the potential for hands-on and applied learning are endless.

The OVC is one of the founding colleges of the University of Guelph, a university consistently ranked the top comprehensive university in Ontario and placed among the top three in Canada by Maclean's Magazine. A national survey of university graduates rated the University of Guelph number one in all but one category, putting it at the top of the list of universities graduates would endorse.

One of five veterinary colleges in Canada, OVC is accredited by the American Veterinary Medical Association, Canadian and American Medical Associations and the Royal College of Veterinary Surgeons of the United Kingdom. OVC grads can be licensed in these countries, giving graduates a spectrum of opportunities.

## APPLICATION INFORMATION

Each year, the Ontario Veterinary College (OVC) accepts up to 15 U.S. and international (non-Canadian) students. This year, you could be one of those students!

International applicants must not hold Canadian citizenship (this includes dual citizenship) or Permanent Resident status. Students can apply as early as the summer after their Sophomore year provided they have a GPA of 3.2 or over and have done the following 8 prerequisite courses:

- 3 Biology
- Genetics
- Biochemistry
- Statistics
- 2 Humanities/Social Sciences

Applicants who receive an offer of admission should be aware that they must meet federal immigration requirements for entry into Canada as a student.

| PREREQUISITES FOR ADMISSION | | |
|---|---|---|
| Course Description | Number of Hours/Credits | Necessity |
| Biology | 9 | Required |
| Biochemistry | 3 | Required |
| Statistics | 3 | Required |
| Genetics | 3 | Required |
| Humanities/Social Science | 6 | Required |

Non-Canadian applicants who have fulfilled the academic requirements for the Doctor of Veterinary Medicine (DVM) program at the Ontario Veterinary College, University of Guelph should apply using the Veterinary Medical College Application Service (VMCAS).

## SUMMARY OF ADMISSIONS PROCEDURES

Checklist for non-Canadians applying to the University of Guelph DVM program

Note: if you hold dual Canadian citizenship you MUST apply as a Canadian.

### Pre-Application

Complete 2 years of university and the 8 prerequisites within full-time semesters.

### Application (October)

Veterinary Medical College Application Service (VMCAS) online application including:

- 3 referee assessments submitted (from 2 veterinarians and 1 professional)
- Background information
- Application fee (to VMCAS)
- The supplemental application form must be submitted separately.
- If you are already attending or have attended the University of Guelph please apply using the Application for Internal Transfer/Readmission Form.

Information is gathered through the Background Information Form (BIF), References, Transcript and GRE scores.

### November

- Academic Background Form with Course Descriptions
- Supplemental fee

You will be assigned a University of Guelph email account with which you can access your WebAdvisor account for updates on your application status.

### December-July

If selected for an interview, you will be contacted by email. Interviews are 45 minutes long with two members of faculty and are usually held at the Ontario Veterinary College in Guelph. Virtual interviews using professional grade video conferencing are offered on a case by case basis.

At the end of your interview you will be provided with a tour of the college led by a current DVM student.

Applicants will then be notified by email and letter of the final decision regarding their application.

*Application directly to the university of Guelph is also available and forms can be obtained by emailing vetmed@uoguelph.ca

If you have questions about the application procedure or a current application in progress, please contact:
Deanna Lundmark, Admission Services
519-824-4120 Ext. 56060.
Entrance Requirements
University

Complete at least two years (4 semesters) of full-time studies in university. Full-time is usually 12 credit hours at a US school.

All prerequisite courses must be completed in acceptable full-time semesters in any year of their university studies. Courses should be completed within a university undergraduate program - courses taken during graduate programs, professional programs, and certificate programs are not acceptable.

Students from the US should take a minimum of 12.00 credit hours per semester. Courses must be taken/studied at the same time to ensure an appropriate work load. Field courses or any courses that are pursued over one semester and credited in another semester do not count towards the latter semester's courses for this purpose.

You can study at any accredited university and take any major that interests you. You can apply to the DVM program in your third year, after finishing two years of university. If accepted, you do not need to finish your four-year degree program and can simply transfer to the DVM.

A course that runs the full year will have the credit weight divided equally and half applied to each of the two semesters the course is taken.

Please note that the GPA from your last two full-time semesters, and the average from your 8 prerequisite courses must both be 3.2 or higher in order for you to be considered further for entry to the DVM program.

*Prerequisite Courses*
3 Biological Sciences (with recommended emphasis on animal biology and one course dealing with cell structure and function)
    Genetics
    Biochemistry
    Statistics
2 Humanities/social sciences (Consider topics such as ethics, logic, critical thinking, determinants of human behaviour and human social interaction.)

*Important Regulations Regarding Acceptable Courses*
The specific course requirements listed below must have been completed at the university level before admission to the Doctor of Veterinary Medicine Program will be considered. Courses do not need to be completed in a designated Pre-Veterinary program.

Courses will not be acceptable if they are repeats of previously passed courses, or if they are taken at the same level or a lower level in a subject area than previously passed courses in the same subject area. This includes courses with significant overlap in content. Students should consider their institution's course sequencing in determining if a course is considered the same level.

The DVM Admissions Committee cannot evaluate Honours, Pass-Fail, and Satisfactory-Unsatisfactory grading systems. Applicants should obtain a numerical or letter grade for all required courses and the grades should be certified by the Registrar of the university attended.

A maximum of TWO acceptable distance education, online courses may be included in a semester. The semester must include a minimum of 12 acceptable credit hours total.

A person's semester/year level is determined by the number of credits that have been completed successfully in his or her degree program plus those that are in progress. Once a person has reached 48 credit hours, he or she is considered a third-year student.

Candidates who hold a non-science bachelor's degree in which they did not take some of the prerequisite courses because they were not part of their program may return to university as part of a non-degree semester(s) to gain the prerequisites for DVM. These courses must be assessed by the University of Guelph Admissions Office for content.

Applicants with a degree who have a documented commitment, such as work or family responsibility, can present their case to the Admission Committee requesting the option of completing their academic requirements on a part-time basis. This should be done before starting the return to classes. See below for the process.

Failure to comply with the course level rules will result in the exclusion of all coursework from the ineligible semester(s) toward a DVM application.

*Course Evaluation Request*
If you are not studying at the University of Guelph, you must submit up to two options for the courses that you want to use as prerequisites for approval prior to application.

Requests must include:

- A transcript of university courses completed to date—a photocopy is fine.

- A list of proposed courses for any future semesters you are planning.

- A list of the eight courses to be presented as prerequisite courses and detailed course descriptions/syllabus for each. You may present one or two choices (no more) for each of the eight. Please be sure to include course codes, titles, and to identify which course is being presented as which prerequisite.

- Your email address and contact information.

Please do not email course evaluation requests. Submit by fax or mail only to:
Deanna Lundmark
Admission Services UC L3
University of Guelph
Guelph, ON N1G 2W1
Fax: 519-766-9481

*Appeals Process / Request to Study the Prerequisites During Part-Time Semesters*
Individuals wishing to appeal decisions related to admissions eligibility may submit a letter detailing their individual circumstance and any letters/documentation of support to:

Chair, Admissions Committee, Ontario Veterinary College
c/o Deanna Lundmark
Admission Services UC L3
University of Guelph
Guelph, ON N1G 2W1
Fax: 519-766-9481

Please note that appeals may take up to two months to process, and submitting an appeal in no way guarantees a positive response.

*Non-academic requirements*

*Veterinary experience*
Veterinary experience may be voluntary or paid, but must be done with a supervising veterinarian in placements such as clinical practice, research laboratories, animal shelters, animal rehabilitation facilities, public health settings or another related industry where a veterinarian is employed.

Although there are no required number of hours needed for application, it is strongly advised that applicants log as many hours as possible. Try working with different species, too, such as swine, cows, horses, exotics, dogs, cats, etc.

Experience within Canada and the USA is recommended.

*Animal experience*
Animal experience includes working with livestock, breeding/showing various species, working in a pet store, equestrian activities and any other animal related hobby/experience where a veterinarian is not always present, or does not supervise you. Animal experience does not include pet ownership. Animals are defined as vertebrates for this purpose.

*Extracurricular experience*
So much of veterinary medicine involves working with people and as part of a team. Jobs and volunteer activities that hone your communication, interpersonal and organizational skills are important. These experiences do not involve animal contact.

*Referee assessments*
Three only confidential referee assessments comprised of an evaluative grid and a letter are required for each DVM applicant.

The referees have to be qualified to give an unbiased, informed and critical assessment of the applicant. Two of the three referees selected must be veterinarians with whom he or she has obtained veterinary and/or animal experience. There is a strong preference for veterinarians from different clinics or workplaces. The goal of having the veterinary references is to have those within the profession assess whether your are a suitable candidate to join that profession, therefore it is important that the referees understand what is required of veterinarians in a Canadian/US context.

None of your references should be from family members, long standing friends, or your colleagues or colleagues of your family, even if they are veterinarians. These are not considered objective sources. Your referees should be individuals who know you in a supervisory or professional context and are able to assess you objectively. Applications from candidates with referee assessments from family, colleagues or friends will not be considered suitable for further consideration and will not be invited for an interview.

Graduate students (those from master's or doctoral degree programs) may request an additional form to highlight their accomplishments while within their graduate program.

*Is a Bachelor's Degree Required?* no

*Is this an International School?* yes

## ESTIMATED TUITION

*Estimated Tuition Resident:* n/a

*Estimated Tuition Contract:* n/a

*Estimated Tuition Non-Resident:* $53,556.88 Canadian Funds

## AVAILABLE SEATS

*Resident:* n/a

*Contract:* n/a

*Non-Resident:* 17

## TEST REQUIREMENTS

GRE general

*VMCAS Participation:* full

*Accepts International Students?* yes

## ADDITIONAL INFORMATION

*Application Deadline:* 10/2/2014

# MASSEY UNIVERSITY

Email Address: vetschool@massey.ac.nz
Website: massey.ac.nz/vetschool

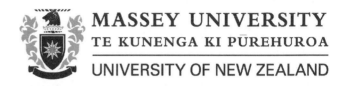

**MASSEY UNIVERSITY**
TE KUNENGA KI PŪREHUROA

UNIVERSITY OF NEW ZEALAND

## SCHOOL DESCRIPTION

The Massey University veterinary program was the first veterinary program to gain AVMA accreditation in the southern hemisphere. The veterinary school accepts up to 24 international students annually with a total class size of 105. The first class of Massey veterinarians graduated in 1967, and since then more than 2,500 veterinarians have graduated and are working around the world.

> The Massey University veterinary school staff are collegial, motivated, highly qualified individuals.

The Massey University veterinary program has an international reputation for providing an excellent veterinary education with a strong science background, a broad knowledge of companion, equine, and production animal health, and a focus on independent thinking and problem-solving skills. The curriculum incorporates practical aspects throughout all years of the degree beginning with animal handling and behaviour in the first post-selection semester through to the final year of the program, which is almost entirely clinically based.

Years 1-4 of the program initially focus on instruction in the core medical sciences tailored for veterinary students to learn normal form and function, and then help the student recognize abnormality, and focus on return to normal through medicine, surgery, health management, diagnostics and treatment of companion and agricultural animal species. A revised curriculum was introduced in 2013 that aims to increase student learning and understanding by integrating topics within

and between years, and introducing problem oriented learning throughout the curriculum. Additionally a greater emphasis has been placed on professional studies, to help enhance student success post-graduation.

The fifth year is a semi-tracked clinically based year. Each student will choose a track from the following options: small animal, production animal, equine or mixed animal, or other areas as approved (i.e. wildlife, research). All tracks share a core of 18 weeks of rotations covering multiple species, then depending on the track a further 7-9 weeks will be prescribed. The student will then have 7-9 weeks where they can choose to do externships (within New Zealand or overseas), or further clinics at Massey University. The semi-tracked, individualized final year curriculum allows students to further explore their area of interest while ensuring wide coverage of the main veterinary species.

The veterinary facilities are of a high international standard, and are currently being expanded and renovated. There are numerous other university-run animal units (dairy, beef, sheep and deer farms, equine blood typing unit, feline unit, large animal teaching unit, etc.) on or adjacent to the Palmerston North campus. The veterinary teaching hospital sees first opinion cases as well as referral cases to provide a balanced clinical experience for the students. The Massey University veterinary school staff are collegial, motivated, highly qualified individuals, many of whom are board certified specialists in their discipline.

The vet school is located in Palmerston North, a student-friendly town of 75,000 in the lower central north island of New Zealand. Nicknamed "student city," Palmerston North offers free bus service to Massey students and is home to numerous cafés, restaurants, bars, theatres, and outdoor recreational activities. Palmerston North is a one-hour flight from Auckland, is conveniently close to west coast beaches, and is just under a two-hour drive to the Hawke's Bay wine region, skiing and snowboarding at Mt Ruapehu and the capital city, Wellington. Renowned for an excellent lifestyle, New Zealand is a great place to study abroad for your AVMA accredited veterinary degree.

## APPLICATION INFORMATION

Specific information (availability, deadlines, fees, and VMCAS participation, the supplemental application and direct application) can be found on the Massey University veterinary school website listed in the contact details above.

US and Canadian residents may apply to Massey University by either:
1. VMCAS and a supplemental Massey University application or
2. Direct application to Massey University.

All other non New Zealand residents are to apply directly to Massey University

*Residency implications:* All non-New Zealand resident students require a student visa, which is easily obtained following an offer of admission into the program. Students must be able to ensure financial support for the duration of their course.

## SUMMARY OF ADMISSIONS PROCEDURES

*Timetable*

*Group 1 (semester 1)*

*Application deadline:* November 1

*Date letters of admission to semester 1 sent:* once completed application received and processed.

*School begins:* late February (semester 1)

*Date acceptances into the veterinary degree program mailed:* early July

*Date veterinary degree program begins:* mid-July (semester 2)

*Group 2*

*VMCAS application deadline:* Thursday, October 2, 2014 1:00 PM Eastern Time (VMCAS application completed online. Supplemental application with all supplementary documents to be received by November 1.)

*Direct applicants:* November 1 (including all supplementary documents)

*Date acceptances mailed:* from late December

*School begins:* mid-July 2014 (semester 2)

*Deposit (to hold Group 2 position):* $NZ 1,500.00

*Deferments:* offers of a place in semester 2 of the program are for a single year only. Deferments are not permitted. Deferments of offers of a place in semester 1 of the program (Group 1 applicants) are permitted.

## EVALUATION CRITERIA

*Group 1*

Weighted GPA (Minimum of a B average across all 4 semester one classes needed to be eligible for selection. Actual GPA for selection is generally higher): 80%

Special Tertiary Admissions Test (STAT) This is the Australian equivalent to the GRE and is held at Massey University in the June examination period at the end of semester one: 20%

*Group 2*

Science GPA: 50%

GRE General Test: 50%

## ENTRANCE REQUIREMENTS

*Course requirements*

*Group 1:* Competitive Selection into Vet School via Semester 1 (10-14 places available)

Group 1 applicants come to Massey University to complete a semester (beginning in late February of each year) of full-time science study (4 classes) at Massey University in order to develop a GPA for selection. Credit will be given where similar classes to the four prerequisite classes have already been completed, and alternate science classes will be chosen by the student.

*Group 2:* Competitive Selection directly into BVSc Semester 2 (10-14 places available)

Applicants are required to have completed at least two full years of full-time, largely science based university education. Applicants need to have passed classes equivalent to the 4 standard Massey University veterinary prerequisite classes:

Massey University Class: Usual classes needed for credit

123.101

Chemistry and Living Systems: General chemistry + Organic chemistry

124.111

Physics for Life Sciences: 1 year of physics

162.101

Biology of Cells (molecular) biology +/- First year biology series

199.101

Biology of Animals: Animal biology / vertebrate zoology

Each of the above classes should include laboratories.

*Required undergraduate GPA:* A minimum science GPA of 3.00 is required to be eligible for selection into the veterinary degree.

*Course completion deadline:*

*Group 1:* not applicable; courses completed in New Zealand.

*Group 2:* all required courses should be completed by the end of the fall semester in the year prior to matriculation (i.e., Fall 2014 for matriculation in 2015).

*Standardized examinations:*

Graduate Record Examination (GRE), general test, is required for Group 2 applicants only. Test scores should be no older than 5 years immediately preceding the application deadline. Scores must be received by the supplemental application deadline.

The STAT-F test is required for Group 1 applicants only. The test will be offered at Massey University in the June examination period. In the uncommon situation that a student sat the STAT-F test elsewhere the deadline for submission of scores would be June 15.

## ADDITIONAL REQUIREMENTS AND CONSIDERATIONS

All VMCAS applicants must complete the supplemental application for Massey University. Your application will not be processed until we have received your supplemental application.

*The supplemental application consists of:*

- A Massey University application for admission as an international student.
- Your GRE score—either a sealed original copy or a copy supplied directly from ETS.
- A letter signed by a veterinarian on his/her clinic letterhead verifying you have completed a minimum of 10 days (80 hours) work experience at their clinic. ELoR's submitted by veterinarians as part of the VMCAS application can be substituted for the signed letter.

Letters of recommendation are not required. A bachelors degree is not a prerequisite requirement for admission into the veterinary degree.

*Is a Bachelor's Degree Required?* no

*Is this an International School?* yes

## ESTIMATED TUITION

*Estimated Tuition Resident:* subsidized

*Estimated Tuition Contract:* 0

*Estimated Tuition Non-Resident:* $NZ 54,600

## AVAILABLE SEATS

*Resident:* 81

*Contract:* 0

*Non-Resident:* 24

## TEST REQUIREMENTS

*Standardized examinations:* Graduate Record Examination (GRE), general test, is required for Group 2 applicants only. Test scores should be no older than 5 years immediately preceding the application.

*VMCAS Participation:* partial

*Accepts International Students?* yes

## ADDITIONAL INFORMATION

*Please note:* the tuition fees are in New Zealand dollars. The actual cost in your currency will depend on the exchange rate at the time of paying tuition fees. The NZD is traditionally lower than the USD and CAD.

*Application Deadline:* 11/1/2014

*VMCAS Deadline:* 10/2/2014

# UNIVERSITY OF MELBOURNE

Admissions Office
The Faculty of Veterinary Science
The University of Melbourne
Corner Park Drive and Flemington Road
Parkville
3010
Victoria
Australia
Tel: + (613) 8344 7357
Fax: + (613) 8344 7374
www.vet.unimelb.edu.au

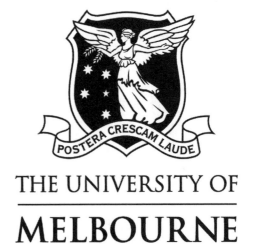

THE UNIVERSITY OF

# MELBOURNE

## SCHOOL DESCRIPTION

The University of Melbourne has a 150-year history of leadership in research, innovation, teaching and learning. As a University of Melbourne student, you will become part of a dynamic collegial environment with a distinctive research edge. Throughout its history the University of Melbourne has educated some of the world's most eminent scientists and researchers and this tradition continues today.

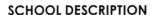

The University of

Melbourne has a

150-year history of

leadership in research,

innovation, teaching

and learning.

The Faculty of Veterinary Science was the very first veterinary school established in Australia, and celebrated its centenary in 2009. It is concentrated on two sites: the city-centre University campus in Parkville and the Werribee campus, where students study in a state-of-the-art teaching hospital designed to support top-class veterinary education in the twenty-first century. Facilities include ten consulting rooms, modern diagnostic capabilities including endoscopy, CT, MRI, image intensification, scintigraphy, on-site diagnostic pathology laboratories and a 24-hour small animal emergency and critical care unit.

The veterinary program is made up of industry-linked learning, practical components and internship opportunities. Students gain experience in animal handling, care and management and undertake professional work experience between semesters and academic years, as well as having hands-on experience throughout the course. The school has strong programs in small animal medicine, equine, dairy cattle, sheep and beef cattle medicine.

The degree is accredited by the American Veterinary Medical Association (AVMA), by the Royal College of Veterinary Surgeons (UK), and by the Australasian Veterinary Boards Council Inc. These accreditations reflect the high quality and international standing of the course and permits graduates of the course to work as veterinarians in a wide range of countries including North America.

Our success has been achieved by insisting on international excellence. Talented people from all over the world come to visit, study and work at the University of Melbourne. At last count, the University's student community of 44,000 included more than 9,800 international students from over 100 countries.

We invite you to join our tradition and discover why staff and students of the highest calibre are attracted to study at the Faculty of Veterinary Science at the University of Melbourne.

## COURSE DURATION, ENTRY ROUTES AND STUDENT NUMBERS

The University of Melbourne offers studies in veterinary education through our professional entry graduate degree; the Doctor of Veterinary Medicine. The four-year degree offers veterinary students the best possible preparation for twenty-first century careers in a rapidly changing and increasingly global workforce. As a result of this change, students can enter the veterinary science program by one of two pathways:

1. Students can apply for entry into the three-year Bachelor of Science degree at the University of Melbourne. After completing prerequisite first and second year subjects,

students will apply for selection to the Veterinary Bioscience specialisation of the Animal Health and Disease major that is offered in the third year of the Bachelor of Science. Students who successfully complete all studies in the Veterinary Bioscience specialisation and who successfully complete the Bachelor of Science overall will have guaranteed entry to the DVM program with 100 points' credit (one year of DVM study).

2. Students can complete a science degree at another institution, and then apply for entry to the DVM at the University of Melbourne. Students will need to have studied at least one semester in each of general or cellular biology and biochemistry within their science degree. Students who follow this pathway will enter the four-year graduate-entry DVM program.

## NUMBER OF INTERNATIONAL STUDENTS THAT WE ACCEPT

We currently accept up to 50 international students from across the globe.

## PREREQUISITES FOR ADMISSION

1. Entrance to the DVM via the Melbourne Bachelor of Science: North American students should refer to the University's international prospectus for up to date details about entrance requirements for the Bachelor of Science by visiting futurestudents .unimelb.edu.au.

2. After completing prerequisite first and second year subjects in the Bachelor of Science, students will be eligible to apply for entry to the Veterinary Bioscience specialisation of the Animal Health and Disease major in third year. Students who successfully complete all studies in the Veterinary Bioscience specialisation will have guaranteed entry into the DVM, with 100 points' credit (one year of study), leaving three years of study in the DVM.

3. Entrance to the DVM as a graduate: Applicants will require a science degree from the University of Melbourne or another institution. Examples of appropriate degrees include Bachelor's degrees with majors in: Agriculture, Animal Science, Biochemistry, Biomedicine, Physiology or Zoology. Prerequisites for entry as a graduate are at least one semester of study in each of general or cellular biology and biochemistry as part of a science degree.

4. There is no standardised test required.

## APPLICATION INFORMATION

International applications will be accepted throughout the year. Applications close in late December, commencing enrolment into the following year, however, this is subject to places still being available. Applicants are advised to apply as soon as possible to avoid disappointment. Applications will be considered as soon as they are received. We recognise the amount of time required by successful applicants to make arrangements for international travel and study and we try to give them as much advance notice as possible.

Students apply via the International Admissions Office at the University of Melbourne. They can choose to apply online, download an application form, apply through one of our overseas representatives or request an undergraduate application form to be posted to them. Visit futurestudents.unimelb.edu.au/info/international.

## TUITION FEES

For information about tuition fees please visit future students.unimelb.edu.au/admissions/fees to access the University's fee tables for international students.

*Application fee:* AUD$100

**Visas:** All non-Australian students require a student visa, which is easily obtained following an offer of admission into our program. More information can be viewed on the website: services.unimelb.edu.au /international/visas/apply.

*Deferments:* Please note that successful applicants may not defer commencement of the DVM. Students can reapply for a start year intake when they are able to commence studies, and the application fee will be waived for international students.

# NATIONAL AUTONOMOUS UNIVERSITY OF MEXICO (UNAM) COLLEGE OF VETERINARY MEDICINE*

Office of Undergraduate Studies (División de Estudios Profesionales)
College of Veterinary Medicine (FMVZ)
Av. Universidad 3000
Circuito Interior
Delegación Coyoacán
México D.F. 04510
Telephone: 56 22 58 80
Webpage: www.fmvz.unam.mx, http://escolar.fmvz.unam.mx
Email: fmvyz@galois.dgae.unam.mx

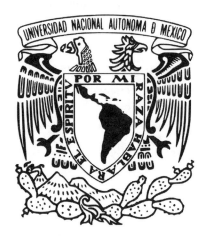

## APPLICATION INFORMATION

Undergraduate admission of new students to the National Autonomous University of Mexico (UNAM) is done through the General Administration Scholar Affairs Direction (DGAE).

The applicants to the College of Veterinary Medicine, students are evaluated in terms of their general academic background, with emphasis on Biology, Chemistry, Physics and Mathematics.

> The University of Melbourne has a 150-year history of leadership in research, innovation, teaching and learning.

There are two annual applications dates: January and April. Information for specific applications dates can be reviewed at www.escolar.unam.mx (the semester starts in August).

Application forms can be found at the same website. The number of available positions is 450, without distinction for Mexican or foreign applicants.

## RESIDENCY IMPLICATIONS

There are no resident implications. All the students have to take the admission test. Recommendation letters are not needed.

## PREREQUISITES FOR ADMISSION

Applicants must have at least a high school average grade of 70%.

Minimum of semesters needed in: mathematics, physics, chemistry, and biology

CURSES (Semesters)

Mathematics (4 semesters)

Physics (4 semesters)

Inorganic and organic chemistry (4 semesters)

Principles of biology and general biology (4 semesters)

Social sciences / humanities (6 semesters)

Electives (2 semesters): selected topics on biology, statistics, morphophysiology or physicochemistry

For students from foreign high schools, beside the admission test, they have to submit all necessary official documents to "Dirección General de Incorporación y Revalidación de Estudios (DGIRE) UNAM". Submission instructions can be found at http://www.dgire.unam.mx/contenido/revalidacion/revalbachc.html.

Foreign students whose primary language is not Spanish will have to do a proficiency Spanish language test.

*Required undergraduate GPA:* It is not necessary

*AP credit policy:* Is not part of the admission requirements

*Course completion deadline:* It is based on the application dates, in January and June.

*Standardized Examinations:* They are not used

*Additional requirements and considerations:* Foreign students must have a good command of the Spanish language

*These pages are for last year's admissions cycle. For updated information, please visit: www.fmvz.unam.mx or http://escolar.fmvz.unam.mx

## SUMMARY OF ADMISSION PROCEDURE

*Timetable*

The next application dates can be checked at www.escolar.unam.mx

*Deposit:* It is not necessary

*Deferments:* Considered on an individual basis, and ordinarily granted for personal reasons, illness, lack of economic resources or other situations beyond the control of the students.

*Evaluation criteria:* Grade of 80% or above in the admission exam.

## 2012–2013 ADMISSIONS SUMMARY

| Number of Applicants | Number of New Entrants |
|---|---|
| 2,742 | 99 (3.6%) |

## EXPENSES FOR THE 2012–2013 ACADEMIC YEAR

(subject to change)

*Tuition and fees:* $2,000 USD per year

# UNIVERSITÉ DE MONTRÉAL

Service de l'admission et du recrutement Université de Montréal
C.P. 6205
Succursale Centre-Ville Montréal Québec H3C 3T5 Canada
Telephone: (514) 343-7076
Webpage: www.medvet.umontreal.ca
Email: saefmv@medvet.umontreal.ca

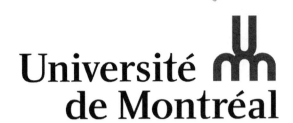

## APPLICATION INFORMATION

*Applications available:* December
    Online: 90$

*Application deadline:* February 1

*Residency implications:* Canadian citizenship or permanent residency in Canada is required.

A total of 90 students are admitted each year.

> A total of 90 students are admitted each year. All lectures are given in French. Examinations must be written in French.

To be considered for admission, one must: a) have completed the above requirements, or b) have completed equivalent studies.

Note: All lectures are given in French. Examinations must be written in French.

The DMV is a 5-year program.

*Condition concerning the knowledge of French:* To be admissible, the candidate must demonstrate that he/she has acquired the minimal level of proficiency in French as required by the chosen program, as established by the University. To this end, the candidate must either:

- succeed the Épreuve uniforme de langue et littérature française of the Ministry of Education of Quebec or;
- obtain a score of at least 785/990 on the International French exam (Test de français international TFI) http://www.etudes.umontreal.ca/programme/doc_prog/section2.pdf.

*Performance Score:* This score is obtained by comparing the student's grade in each course with the class average.

*Course completion deadline:* The applicant must have completed all prerequisites at the time of application.

*Additional considerations (in order of importance)*
    1. Academic record
    2. Admission test

## SUMMARY OF ADMISSION PROCEDURE

*Timetable*

*Application deadline:* February 1

*Interviews:* beginning of May

*Notification of acceptance:* end of May, early June

*Fall semester begins:* end of August

*Deposit (to hold place in class):* 200 $C

| Evaluation criteria | % |
| --- | --- |
| Performance score | 80 |
| Interview | 20 |

## ESTIMATED EXPENSES FOR THE 2011–2012 ACADEMIC YEAR

*Tuition and fees:* 72.26 $C per credit for residents of Quebec (approx. 45 per year)

195.27 $ per credit for Canadian non-residents of Quebec

# FOURTH-YEAR PROFILE: SAMANTHA VITALE

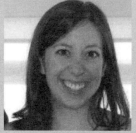

**What has been your favorite thing about attending veterinary school so far?**
I have enjoyed clinics and externships very much. We have a great curriculum that allows for two years of clinical experience, which has been a great learning experience and allows us to finally put all of our hard work into practice.

**What advice do you have for prospective veterinary school applicants?**
Live your life first! I have focused on becoming a veterinarian since I was fifteen, which I don't regret, because I cannot wait to finally be a veterinarian. While I would encourage everyone to study hard and get as much veterinary experience as possible to boost their résumé, I would also encourage them to pursue other passions while they have the chance. Study abroad, get a job outside of the veterinary industry, take classes that have nothing to do with your major—just live. This is a wonderful profession, but there is a beautiful world outside of that. Sometimes, if you get too focused on a goal, you can lose sight of that.

**What are your short-term and long-term goals?**
Short term I am hoping to get a small animal rotating internship and then a residency in neurology. Long-term I would like to work in large referral practice and have a family.

**What extracurricular activities have you been involved in during veterinary school?**
I served as president of the student chapter of the Disaster Animal Response Team and as a member of the MSU chapter of the Student American Veterinary Medical Association, the MSU CVM Curriculum Committee, the Veterinary Business Management Association, and the Mississippi Animal Response Team. I have also served as the student representative for Bayer Animal Health, the North American Veterinary Conference, and VCA.

**What was the biggest challenge you faced during veterinary school?**
Second semester of sophomore year was our toughest course load. It was difficult to stay motivated at the end of that marathon of studying, but it was worth it.

**Do you plan to practice veterinary medicine after graduating from veterinary school?**
Yes, I hope to become boarded in neurology, and I plan to work in private practice for the duration of my career.

**What advice do you have for other students who are currently in veterinary school?**
Study hard and be flexible about your goals. You may discover that you want to pursue a different path than you initially thought, so focus on making connections and learning as much as you can.

**Why do you want to be a veterinarian?**
I cannot remember every wanting to do anything else. It is just a part of who I am.

# MURDOCH UNIVERSITY

Email Address: international@murdoch.edu.au
Website: http://www.murdoch.edu.au/School-of-Veterinary-and-Life-Sciences/

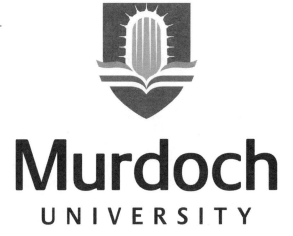

## SCHOOL DESCRIPTION

Western Australia is known for its brilliant blue skies, warm sunny climate and white sandy beaches. It is a land blessed with some of the world's most precious natural phenomena including the dolphins of Monkey Mia, the 350-million-year-old Bungle Bungle range and the towering karri forests of the South West. Sophisticated yet uncomplicated, the lifestyle for the residents of Perth is relaxed and focuses on the outdoors.

There are wineries, beaches, bushland, and unique wildlife within easy reach of the city, and a cosmopolitan mix of cafes, restaurants, pubs and thriving nightlife in the city centre.

> Veterinary students learn in a true practice atmosphere with the final year of study devoted entirely to clinical exposure.

Veterinary students from Murdoch graduate with a double degree (Bachelor of Science and Bachelor of Veterinary Medicine and Surgery) after one year of general science and 5 years of veterinary specific units. The course is designed to impart the knowledge and skills necessary for the diagnosis, treatment and prevention of disease and production problems in pets, farm animals, wildlife and laboratory animals. Veterinary students learn in a true practice atmosphere with the final year of study lecture-free and devoted entirely to clinical exposure, including time spent at Perth Zoo. Murdoch students have access to state-of-the art facilities, all on the one campus, including a 24-hour emergency clinic, large and small animal practices, a well-stocked farm and an equine hospital as well as production animal and equine ambulatory ser-

vices. The thriving practices have very busy caseloads, serviced by many specialist clinicians, so that students can gain extensive experience.

The curriculum keeps Murdoch at the forefront of veterinary education worldwide. This curriculum allows more time for students to develop areas of special interest through non-core rotations, special topics, externships and extramural experience. A Veterinary Professional Life stream is integrated throughout the course to assist students in their transition to future careers in veterinary science and provides a strong focus for developing professional life skills within the veterinary profession. An Animal Systems stream will allow strengthening and integration of animal production, animal ethics, animal welfare, animal behaviour, biosecurity and veterinary public health throughout the veterinary program.

The veterinary science degree is accredited by the American Veterinary Medical Association (AVMA), the Royal College of Veterinary Surgeons (UK), and the Australian Veterinary Boards Council. Completing your Veterinary Science degree Murdoch saves you years of study, and potentially thousands of dollars; this is because with the correct preparation, the 5 years of veterinary specific tuition can be entered into after only one year of tertiary study in general biological science. Once you have finished your degree at Murdoch, you are eligible to sit your exams with the AVMA just as you would if you completed your studies in North America.

## APPLICATION INFORMATION

For specific information (availability, deadlines, fees, and VMCAS participation), please refer to the contact information listed above.

All non-residents require a student visa, which is easily obtained following an offer of admission into the veterinary course. Applicants whose first language is not English must demonstrate competency in the English language.

## SUMMARY OF ADMISSIONS PROCEDURES

*Timetable*

There are four application deadlines each year, which are: March 31, June 30, September 30 and November 30.

*School begins:* mid-February

Some candidates may be eligible to begin in early August.

*VMCAS application deadline:* not applicable. Students are to apply direct via Murdoch. Application form can be found at http://www.murdoch.edu.au/Future -students/International-students/Applying-to-Murdoch /Application-forms/

*Deposit to hold a position:* $1,000 AUD payable upon acceptance of offer

## ENTRANCE REQUIREMENTS

Students that have completed one or more years of tertiary study are eligible to apply for entry into the five year Veterinary course. Your first year of tertiary study must include units in Chemistry, Cell Function/Biology, introductory Anatomy and Physiology, and Statistics.

Applications are also accepted from school leavers, with high achievers offered a place in the first general science year at Murdoch with a guaranteed progression into the veterinary specific course, provided they pass all that first year.

Other applicants will be formally selected from those who have successfully completed one year or more of formal tertiary study, including the prerequisite units listed above. Applicants are required to supply with the application form a typed Personal Statement of up to 500 words to which should be attached documents such as curriculum vitae and references, and which should out-line:

Why you wish to become a Veterinarian;

How you consider your past study and experience to date will assist you to succeed in the veterinary course and as a Veterinarian.

If you have any fails/late withdrawals in your post-secondary/tertiary study, you should explain the circumstances for your poor performance and why those circumstances will not apply to your Murdoch studies. You should aim to demonstrate your motivation and preparation for veterinary science.

Assessment of the application will be based on the academic standard achieved in all previous tertiary study, the personal statement, and evidence of recent veterinary and animal related experience. Depending on whether an applicant has satisfied the prerequisites, an offer will be made directly into the veterinary specific part of the course. If not, an offer will be made into the general first year with an assured progression into the veterinary course after successful completion of that year.

*Deferments:* considered on merit

*Is a Bachelor's Degree Required?* no

*Is this an International School?* yes

## ESTIMATED TUITION

*Estimated Tuition Resident:* n/a

*Estimated Tuition Contract:* 0

*Estimated Tuition Non-Resident:* A$40,600 to $57,000 pa

## AVAILABLE SEATS

*Resident:* 0

*Contract:* 0

*Non-Resident:* 45 non-resident

*VMCAS Participation:* non-VMCAS

*Accepts International Students?* yes

## ADDITIONAL INFORMATION

*Application Deadline:* 11/30/2014

# UNIVERSITY OF PRINCE EDWARD ISLAND

Email Address: registrar@upei.ca
Website: http://www.upei.ca/registrar/

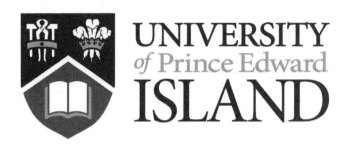

## SCHOOL DESCRIPTION

The Atlantic Veterinary College (AVC), one of the newest colleges of veterinary medicine in North America, opened in 1986 and is fully accredited by the American Veterinary Medical Association, the Canadian Veterinary Medical Association, and the Royal College of Veterinary Surgeons (UK).

Centrally located on Canada's eastern seaboard (650 miles northeast of Boston), the Atlantic Veterinary College makes its home in a beautiful island setting in Charlottetown, Prince Edward Island. With a population of 138,000, which jumps to over a million during the summer tourist season, the community enjoys a small-town lifestyle that boasts the amenities of larger cities, including dining and theatre. Residents also enjoy outdoor activities, such as golfing, cycling, sailing, and cross-country skiing.

> The University of Prince Edward Island is a completely integrated teaching, research, and service facility.

The college is a completely integrated teaching, research, and service facility. The four-story complex contains the veterinary teaching hospital, diagnostic services, fish health unit, farm services, postmortem services, animal barns, laboratories, classrooms, computer and audio-visual facilities, offices, cafeteria, and study areas.

Prince Edward Island is a scenic province with a wide variety of dairy, beef, hog, sheep, horse, and fish farms. The combination and variety of animal and fish farms have allowed AVC to develop a special expertise in fish health, aquaculture, and population medicine.

## APPLICATION INFORMATION

For specific application information (availability, deadlines, fees, and VMCAS participation), please refer to the contact information listed above.

*Residency implications:* Atlantic Veterinary College contracts with New Brunswick (13), Newfoundland (3), Nova Scotia (16), and the home province P.E.I. (10). International students are admitted on a noncontract basis (up to 21).

## SUMMARY OF ADMISSIONS PROCEDURES

*Timetable*

*VMCAS application deadline:* Tuesday, October 2, 2014 1:00 PM Eastern Time

*New Supplementary Application deadline date:* October 2, 2014 (same deadline as VMCAS)

*Date interviews are held:* January–February

*Date acceptances mailed:* January–March

*School begins:* late August; registration, early September

*Deposit (to hold place in class):* 500.00 $C

*Deferments:* are considered on a case-by-case basis.

## EVALUATION CRITERIA

Academic credentials including the GRE are evaluated by the Registrar's Office. Other criteria and activities are evaluated by the admissions committee through an interview process, and the supplementary application.

% weight
Academic ability 55%
Noncognitive ability 35%
Veterinary experience 10%

## ENTRANCE REQUIREMENTS

*Required undergraduate GPA:* no minimum stated (under review as stated above); mean cumulative GPA of most recent entering class is 3.70 on a 4.00 scale.

*AP and IB credit policy:* a maximum of 6 credits accepted.

*Is a Bachelor's Degree Required?* no

*Is this an International School?* yes

## ESTIMATED TUITION

*Estimated Tuition Resident:* $12,601.00 Can (approx)

*Estimated Tuition Contract:* $12,601.00 Can (approx)

*Estimated Tuition Non-Resident:* $55,126.00 Can (approx)

## AVAILABLE SEATS

*Resident:* 10

*Contract:* 32

*Non-Resident:* 20

## TEST REQUIREMENTS

*Standardized examinations:* Graduate Record Examination (GRE) If a student's native language or language of prior education is not English, then the student will be required to submit an acceptable English Proficiency Test score.

*VMCAS Participation:* full

*Accepts International Students?* yes

## ADDITIONAL INFORMATION

*Application Deadline:* 10/2/2014

# UNIVERSITY OF QUEENSLAND

School of Veterinary Sciences
The University of Queensland
Gatton Queensland, 4343
Australia
Tel: + 61 (7) 5460 1834
Fax: + 61 (7) 5460 1922
Email Address: vetenquiries@uq.edu.au
Website: www.uq.edu.au/vetschool

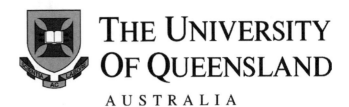

AUSTRALIA

## SCHOOL DESCRIPTION

The University of Queensland's (UQ) School of Veterinary Science is located near the town of Gatton, approximately 40 miles west of Brisbane, Queensland, Australia. The campus has a rural atmosphere, while being no more than an hour's drive from major urban and tourism centers of Brisbane, the Gold Coast and Toowoomba.

Since its first intake of students in 1936, The UQ School of Veterinary Science has been recognized for a sustained record of excellence in teaching and learning across the veterinary disciplines and the quality of its research. The diverse group of academic and clinical staff in the School have made major contributions to tropical/subtropical animal health and medicine to benefit farm and companion animals, their owners and industry sectors.

> The world-class facilities and highly-trained staff ensures the highest standard of veterinary training.

Following the relocation to the UQ Gatton Campus in 2010, the School's values remain strongly orientated towards maintaining the strong sense of community for which the school is renowned. With new facilities, and an ambitious recruitment program that has attracted an excellent cohort of staff, UQ has backed the School to outperform standards of education in Australasia, a performance reflecting UQ's global ranking in the top 100 university. The world-class facilities and highly-trained staff ensure the School exceeds international accreditation guidelines, ensuring the highest standard of veterinary training. We anticipate a DVM program with enhanced admissions criteria will be established at UQ within the next few years.

Upon its relocation to the UQ Gatton Campus, the School commissioned four new buildings and, in addition to existing facilities, now comprises the Veterinary Teaching Laboratories, Clinical Studies Centre, Veterinary Science Building and the Veterinary Medical Centre (Equine and Companion Animal Hospitals) complete with the latest instrumentation for diagnostic imaging and surgical techniques. The combination of the School of Veterinary Science, and the Queensland Animal Science Precinct, makes the Gatton campus the most comprehensive animal research and training center in Australia.

The curriculum of the School of Veterinary Sciences is a 10-semester 5 year program that runs from February to November in each year. The first year provides core foundational training in biological sciences, with emphases on animal biology, biochemistry, cellular physiology, anatomy and professional studies. In the second and third years, the emphasis becomes the understanding of diseases, and their causation, diagnosis, treatment and prevention. In the fourth year, a strong clinical focus is provided, which is then reinforced in fifth year through 32 weeks of core and elective clinical rotations, both in the Veterinary Medical Centre and in off-campus practices. A strong commitment to research training in veterinary sciences is provided through clinical research electives. The School of Veterinary Science has outstanding teaching and research programs encompassing all aspects of veterinary science. The School's research strengths lie in biosecurity and infectious diseases, genetics, medicine, nutrition, Australian wildlife, farm animal and equine medicine, production and reproduction.

## APPLICATION INFORMATION

For specific information on application for a place in the program, please refer to the Undergraduate Prospectus of the University of Queensland Faculty of Science, which is updated annually (http://www.science.uq.edu.au/prospectus).

The school enrolls approximately 120 students annually, of which 40 seats are held for nonresident students. Nonresident students must hold a student visa for the duration of their studies.

## SUMMARY OF ADMISSIONS PROCEDURES

There are no specific interviews for international applicants. UQ is moving towards introducing a graduate-entry DVM program in the next few years. This program will have enhanced admissions criteria.

Nonresident applicants for the program at UQ can submit an application directly to the University or through one of UQ's authorized International Education Representatives (http://www.uq.edu.au/international-students/international-educational-representatives).

Resident students or international students studying in Australia apply for entry through the Queensland Tertiary Admissions Center (http://www.qtac.edu.au).

Successful applicants can apply to defer for one year after receiving an offer of a seat in the program.

*Is a Bachelor's Degree Required?* no

*Is this an International School?* yes

## ESTIMATED TUITION

Estimated Tuition Resident: For information about fees for resident students, please visit www.uq.edu.au/study/ to access the University's fee tables for domestic students.

Estimated Tuition Non-Resident (International): For information about tuition fees please visit http://www.uq.edu.au/international-students/ to access the University's fee tables for international students. Full-time enrolment consists of 16 units per annum or 80 units for the veterinary program.

## AVAILABLE SEATS

*Resident:* 80

*Non–Resident (International):* 40

*VMCAS Participation:* non-VMCAS

*Accepts International Students?* yes

## APPLICATION DEADLINE

Nonresident applicants are eligible to participate in Streamlined Visa Processing. It is recommended that nonresident students applications to UQ by November 30 in the year preceding entry.

# ROSS UNIVERSITY SCHOOL OF VETERINARY MEDICINE

Email Address: Admissions@RossU.edu
Website: www.RossU.edu

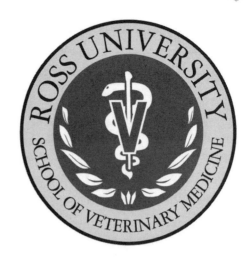

## SCHOOL DESCRIPTION

Located in St. Kitts, West Indies, Ross University School of Veterinary Medicine (RUSVM) offers an American Veterinary Medical Association (AVMA)-accredited* veterinary program focused on educating tomorrow's leaders and discoverers in veterinary medicine. RUSVM is dedicated to providing academic excellence for students as the foundation for becoming sought-after, practice-ready veterinarians for North America and beyond, and has over 3,000 graduates who are successfully practicing veterinary medicine across the US and Canada.

> Ross University's faculty share a passion for educating the veterinarians of tomorrow.

The seven-semester pre-clinical curriculum is enhanced by hands-on clinical experience to help prepare students for the final year of clinical training at one of RUSVM's affiliated veterinary schools in the United States. RUSVM's faculty have outstanding credentials in teaching and research and share a passion for educating the veterinarians of tomorrow. RUSVM operates on a three-semester per year calendar.

Each semester is 15 full academic weeks, including final exams. RUSVM graduates are eligible to practice veterinary medicine in all 50 States, Canada and Puerto Rico upon completion of the requisite licensing requirements. RUSVM students who are U.S. citizens/permanent residents and meet the Department of Education's qualifying criteria may be eligible for Federal Stafford Loans and Federal Graduate PLUS Loans.

## APPLICATION INFORMATION

- Students can apply through VMCAS or directly through RUSVM.

- Evaluation Criteria:

- Undergraduate cumulative grade point average (GPA)

- GPA in required pre-veterinary coursework

- Advanced science courses (Cell Biology, Genetics, Microbiology, Anatomy and Physiology, etc.)

- Graduate Record Examination (GRE) scores

- Personal essay

- Letters of recommendation from academic and/or professional references (at least one letter should be from a veterinarian)

- Extracurricular activities and accomplishments

- Personal qualities

- Personal interview

- Record of Veterinary Profession experience (working with animals or veterinary research) - at least 150 hours

*RUSVM's Doctor of Veterinary Medicine degree program has limited accreditation status from the AVMA COE. AVMA Council on Education · Phone: 800.248.2862 · www.avma.org

## SUMMARY OF ADMISSIONS PROCEDURES

*Timetable (for VMCAS applications)*

*Application deadline:* October 2, 2014; 1:00 PM Eastern Time

*Date interviews are held:* Year-round

*Date acceptances mailed:* As soon as possible after the interview

*School begins:* Three start dates per year: September, January and May

## TIMETABLE

*Application deadline:* None; rolling admissions

*Date interviews are held:* Year-round

*Date acceptances mailed:* As soon as possible after the interview

*School begins:* Three start dates per year: September, January and May

*Deposit (to hold place in class):* $1,000.00

*Deferments:* Considered

## ENTRANCE REQUIREMENTS

To be considered for review by the admission committee the applicant must complete at least 48 credits of college work.

*Course completion deadline:* Required courses must be completed prior to enrollment.

*AP credit policy:* Must appear on official college transcripts.

*Standardized Examinations:* Results of the Graduate Record Examination (GRE) are required.

*English Language Proficiency:* Applicants presenting fewer than 60 upper division credits from an English language college or university must provide the official record of the scores for the Test of English as a Foreign Language (TOEFL). The minimum acceptable score is 550 on the paper-based test, or 213 on the computer-based test.

*Is a Bachelor's Degree Required?* no

*Is this an International School?* yes

## ESTIMATED TUITION

*Estimated Tuition Resident:* 0

*Estimated Tuition Contract:* 0

*Estimated Tuition Non-Resident:* $17,725 per semester

## AVAILABLE SEATS

*Resident:* 0

*Contract:* 0

*Non-Resident:* PENDING

## TEST REQUIREMENTS

Results of the Graduate Record Examination (GRE) are required.

*English Language Proficiency:* Applicants presenting fewer than 60 upper division credits from an English language college or university must provide the official record of the scores for the Test of English as a Foreign Language (TOEFL). The minimum acceptable score is 550 on the paper-based test, or 213 on the computer-based test.

*VMCAS Participation:* partial

*Accepts International Students?* yes

## ADDITIONAL INFORMATION

*Application Deadline:* 10/2/2014

# ROYAL VETERINARY COLLEGE

Royal Veterinary College
University of London
Email Address: admissions@rvc.ac.uk
Website: http://www.rvc.ac.uk/

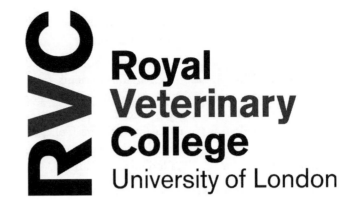

## SCHOOL DESCRIPTION

The RVC has a successful record of training North American students and can count several hundred American and Canadian graduates as alumni. Founded in 1791, the RVC was the first veterinary school in the UK, and the driving force behind the establishment of the nation's veterinary profession. The first four students were admitted in January 1792, and ever since the College has been at the forefront of teaching and research in veterinary and allied sciences. The RVC was the first Veterinary School to submit a woman for membership to the Royal College of Veterinary Surgeons; become an independent veterinary school within a federal university; be accredited by the American Veterinary Medical Association; introduce a degree in Veterinary Nursing; and establish a Centre for Lifelong and Independent Veterinary Education. Today, first-class teaching and research staff, experienced in a wide range of disciplines and skills, help talented students to exploit state-of-the-art clinical facilities and laboratories to the full, maintaining the RVC's long, proud tradition of making seminal contributions to both the animal and human sciences.

> The Royal Veterinary College is at the forefront of teaching and research in veterinary and allied sciences.

We have one campus near Kings Cross/Camden Town, in central London (the London Campus) and one located close to the outskirts of London on a 575-acre site near Potters Bar (the Hertfordshire Campus). Both offer a friendly and supportive environment and excellent facilities for teaching and learning. The London Campus boasts newly refurbished research laboratories, and extensive library, an anatomy museum, the London Bioscience Innovation Centre and the Beaumont-Sainsbury Animal Hospital. Accommodation, a fitness room, a refectory and a bar, and a new social learning space including a cafe are also on site and the clubs, bars, restaurants and theatres of Camden and London's West End are easily accessed on foot or by public transport. A twenty-minute walk from the London Campus is the University of London whose collegiate structure incorporates the RVC. Here in the capital's university quarter, you will find some of the nation's greatest educational and research facilities.

The Hertfordshire Campus is our main clinical campus with three state-of-the-art teaching hospitals on site including the largest veterinary-referral hospital in Europe. Located in rural countryside near Potters Bar, it is a 20 minute train journey from London's Kings Cross station and comprises lecture theatres, laboratories, a Learning Resources Centre (providing superb IT resources and teaching and library facilities), a Clinical Skills Centre and student housing, a refectory, sports fields, and a student-run bar. In addition to the modern journals and textbooks you will find in our libraries, the RVC has one of the best collections of old veterinary books in the world. The RVC has invested heavily in the Hertfordshire Campus in recent years, developing a new Student Village with over 190 bedrooms, a new refectory for both staff and students, a state-of-the-art Teaching and Research Centre and a world-class Equine Hospital. Our working-farm is also located at this campus.

Places in RVC halls of residence are available and students from overseas are given priority. The College has a number of dedicated staff who provide academic and pastoral support to students throughout the course, and we have an active and welcoming student community.

145

## APPLICATION INFORMATION

For specific application information (availability, deadlines, fees and VMCAS participation), please refer to our website at http://www.rvc.ac.uk/Undergraduate/International/Country/NorthAmerica.cfm.

*Residency implications:* The UK government introduced a points-based immigration system for students from non-EU countries who wish to study in the UK. For further information on entry to the UK, please refer to http://www.ukvisas.gov.uk/en/ and to the College's web site. Students must also be able to ensure adequate financial support for the duration of their course.

## SUMMARY OF ADMISSIONS PROCEDURES

*Timetable*

*VMCAS application deadline:* Tuesday, October 2, 2014 1:00 PM Eastern Time

*Immediate offers which do not require an interview are made to exceptional candidates:* November/December

*Interview dates are arranged:* October-December

*Date interviews are held:* January/February (held in the U.S.)

*Date acceptances mailed:* February/March

*School begins:* September

*Transcripts:* All transcripts to VMCAS by 1 September 2014 and fall transcripts to VMCAS by 1 February 2015

*Deposit (to hold place in class):* £1,000 sterling

*Deferments:* may be considered in exceptional circumstances.

## EVALUATION CRITERIA

Academic performance
Animal/veterinary experience
Interview (in most cases)
References/evaluations (minimum 2 required—one from academic science source and one from a veterinary surgeon who you have worked with)
Personal statement

## ENTRANCE REQUIREMENTS

*Course requirements*

VMCAS applicants are normally final year or recent university graduates although students with two years pre-vet will be considered. We will also consider High School students studying AP or the International Baccalaureate. These students apply through UCAS (see our website at http://www.rvc.ac.uk/Undergraduate/International/Country/NorthAmerica.cfm#Applying). Science graduates or applicants in the final year of a science based degree with the prerequisites may be considered for our 4 year accelerated course. Applicants who are unsuccessful in gaining a place

on the four year programme may be considered for our five year programme. Subjects must include Organic Chemistry with lab, Biochemistry, Mathematics or Statistics, Principles of Biology, Physics with lab, General Biology, Animal Biology, or Zoology all with lab. As a minimum we require 8 semester credits in Organic Chemistry and Principles of Biology, General Biology, Animal Biology or Zoology and 4 semester credits in Biochemistry, Physics with Laboratory and Mathematics/Statistics (Algebra is acceptable). It is also recommended that students take General Chemistry or Fundamentals of Chemistry.

*Required undergraduate GPA:* 3.40 or higher preferred (on 4.0 point scale).

*AP credit policy:* not applicable for graduate applicants.

*Course completion deadline:* all required courses should be completed by July of the year of admissions.

*Standardized examinations:* GRE General test required and must be sent to the College by 2 October. RVC institution code is 3207.

## ADDITIONAL REQUIREMENTS AND CONSIDERATIONS

Applicants are also expected to have gained significant relevant work experience of handling animals. This should include work in veterinary practice and where possible other animal establishments.

*Supplemental Application:* not required

*Is a Bachelor's Degree Required?* no

*Is this an International School?* yes

## ESTIMATED TUITION

*Estimated Tuition Resident:* pending, see our website for further information

*Estimated Tuition Contract:* none

*Estimated Tuition Non-Resident:* pending, see our website for further information

## AVAILABLE SEATS

*Resident:* tbc

*Contract:* none

*Non-Resident:* tbc

## TEST REQUIREMENTS

*Standardized examinations:* GRE General test required and to be submitted to the RVC by 2 October. RVC institution code is 3207.

*VMCAS Participation:* partial

*Accepts International Students?* yes

## ADDITIONAL INFORMATION

*Application Deadline:* 10/2/2014

# UNIVERSITY OF SASKATCHEWAN
# WESTERN COLLEGE OF VETERINARY MEDICINE

Email Address: wcvm.admissions@usask.ca
Website: http://www.usask.ca/wcvm

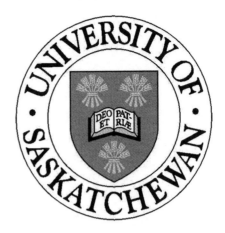

## SCHOOL DESCRIPTION

The Western College of Veterinary Medicine is located in the city of Saskatoon, which has a population of about 265,000 and is the major urban center in central Saskatchewan. The city is also the major commercial center for central and northern Saskatchewan and is served by 2 national airlines with direct connections to all major centers in Canada.

The Western College of Veterinary Medicine is one of the few veterinary colleges where all health sciences and agriculture are offered on the same campus. The college is devoted to undergraduate education and has a reputation in Canada and in the north-western United States for educating veterinarians who are well-rounded in general veterinary medicine and have good practical backgrounds. It has one of the best field-service caseloads in North America.

> The Western College of Veterinary Medicine has one of the best field-service caseloads in North America.

## APPLICATION INFORMATION

For specific application information (availability, deadlines, fees, and VMCAS participation), please refer to the contact information listed above.

*Residency implications:* Currently, 78 students are selected for quota positions from Alberta, British Columbia, Manitoba, Saskatchewan, and the Yukon, Nunavut, and Northwest Territories. Special consideration is given to self identified individuals of aboriginal origin. Residents of foreign countries are not considered.

## SUMMARY OF ADMISSIONS PROCEDURES

*Timetable*

*Application deadline:* December 1

*Reference deadline:* February 15

*Date interviews are held:* May-June

*Date acceptances mailed:* on or before July 1

*School begins:* late August

*Deposit (to hold place in class):* none required.

*Deferments:* not considered.

## EVALUATION CRITERIA

The 3-part admission procedure consists of an assessment of academic ability, a personal interview, and an overall assessment of the application file.

% weight

Grades 60%

Interview* 40%

* Interview selection is based entirely on academic performance.

## ENTRANCE REQUIREMENTS

*Required undergraduate GPA:* a minimum cumulative average of 75% is required.

*Course completion deadline:* prerequisite courses must be completed by the time of entry into the program.

*Standardized examinations:* none required.

## PREREQUISITES FOR ADMISSION

| Course Description | Number of Hours/Credits | Necessity |
|---|:---:|:---:|
| English | 6 | Required |
| Physics | 3 | Required |
| Biology | 6 | Required |
| Genetics | 3 | Required |
| Introductory Chemistry | 6 | Required |
| Organic Chemistry | 3 | Required |
| Mathematics or Statistics | 6 | Required |
| Biochemistry | 3 | Required |
| Microbiology | 3 | Required |
| Electives | 21 | Required |

*Reference Forms:* Two required—one from a veterinarian and one from an individual with an agricultural- or animal-related background.

*Additional Requirements/Information:* Space is provided on the application form to nominate referees to support the application. Referees will be contacted directly and asked to complete the reference form online.

## ADDITIONAL REQUIREMENTS AND CONSIDERATIONS

Animal/veterinary work experience, motivation, and knowledge

Maturity

Leadership

Communication skills

*Is a Bachelor's Degree Required?* no

*Is this an International School?* yes

## ESTIMATED TUITION

*Estimated Tuition Resident:* $8,254.06 $C

*Estimated Tuition Contract:* $8,254.06 $C

*Estimated Tuition Non-Resident:* $8,254.06 $C

## AVAILABLE SEATS

*Resident:* 20

*Contract:* 57

*Non-Resident:* 1

## TEST REQUIREMENTS

None

*VMCAS Participation:* non-VMCAS

*Accepts International Students?* yes

## ADDITIONAL INFORMATION

*Application Deadline:* 12/1/2014

# ST. GEORGE'S UNIVERSITY

Email Address: SGUEnrolment@sgu.edu
Website: http://www.sgu.edu

St. George's University

## SCHOOL DESCRIPTION

Having received full accreditation by the AVMA COE in 2011, St. George's University School of Veterinary Medicine is proud of its academic excellence exemplified by its breadth of highly regarded education, unprecedented student support services, and internationally recognized faculty. The core mission of the University is creating excellent academic programs within an international setting where students and faculty are actively recruited from around the world. St. Georges University has drawn faculty and students from over 140 countries, assembling a diverse community of disparate cultural and educational backgrounds.

> SGU prepares its students for leadership, life-long success and service in a constantly changing world.

Located on the southwest corner of the Caribbean island of Grenada, St. George's shoreline location offers its growing student body a serene environment in which to live, learn and create a worldwide network of friends and colleagues. Along with St. George's state-of-the-art facilities, complete with a large animal facility and, marine station, and the SGU Small Animal Clinic, St. George's University School of Veterinary Medicine prepares its students for leadership, life-long success and service in a constantly changing world.

Over 6,000 students from throughout the world are enrolled in the University's School of Medicine, School of Veterinary Medicine, School of Arts and Sciences or graduate programs which include a CEPH-accredited MPH and MBA program. SGU students also benefit from world-renowned international academic partnerships with universities, hospitals and other educational and scientific institutions.

The veterinary medical program is delivered with a number of entry options: the seven-, six- and five-year programs which begin with the preveterinary medical sciences and an option to enter directly into the four-year veterinary medical program. This enables students flexible entry points depending upon their academic backgrounds. Students accepted into the preveterinary medical sciences are placed in the appropriate program option (either the seven-, six or five-year program track) according to their academic background and are enrolled in the veterinary medical program for five to seven years. Applicants accepted directly into the veterinary medical sciences generally complete the program in four years.

The DVM program is conducted on the University's main campus on the True Blue peninsula of Grenada, West Indies, except for the final year which is the clinical year spent at an affiliated AVMA-accredited School of Veterinary Medicine. These schools are located in the United States, Canada, United Kingdom, Ireland, and Australia.

## APPLICATION INFORMATION

As a member of the Association of American Veterinary Medical Colleges (AAVMC) the School of Veterinary Medicine participates in the AAVMC's centralized Veterinary Medical College Application Service (VMCAS). Aspiring veterinary medical students have the option of applying to the August 2015 or January 2016 entering class through the VMCAS 2015 application cycle. Candidates who intend to apply to veterinary schools through VMCAS can include St.

| PREREQUISITES FOR ADMISSION | | |
| --- | --- | --- |
| Course Description | Number of Hours/Credits | Necessity |
| General Biology or Zoology with Lab | 8 | Required |
| Inorganic Chemistry (general or Physical) with lab | 8 | Required |
| Organic Chemistry with lab | 4 | Required |
| Biochemistry | 3 | Required |
| Genetics | 3 | Required |
| Physics with lab | 4 | Required |
| Calculus, Computer Science or Statistics | 3 | Required |
| English | 3 | Required |

George's University as a designated school and follow the instructions for the SGU supplemental application. To learn more or apply go to aavmc.org/Students-Applicants-and-Advisors/Veterinary-Medical-College-Application-Service.

Applicants who designate St. George's University on the electronic VMCAS application are required to complete a supplemental application. This supplemental application consists of several questions and an essay and is to be completed following submission of the VMCAS application. There is no additional application fee for the supplemental application.

If you are not applying through VMCAS, we encourage you to apply online and track your application status through Self-Service Admission. As an alternative, you can still download a paper copy to print and complete manually.

## SUMMARY OF ADMISSIONS PROCEDURES

*Application Deadlines for August and January Matriculation:* The Committee on Admission utilizes a rolling admission policy in the School of Veterinary Medicine; therefore, applications are accepted and reviewed on an ongoing basis. The final deadline for receipt of direct (non-VMCAS) applications and all supporting documentation is June 15 of the current year for the August class, and November 15 of the preceding year for the January class. Prospective candidates should note that the entering classes are highly competitive and those applications completed early have the advantage of being reviewed at the beginning of the admission process. The time necessary to secure official transcripts, standardized test scores, and letters of recommendation should be taken into consideration. The Committee reserves the right to defer an application to the following semester if there are no available seats.

The Office of Admission will acknowledge receipt of a candidate's application within two weeks of its arrival. A candidate will be informed of any required supporting documents missing at that time. Within one month after receipt of all application materials, a candidate will receive notice that the application is complete and being reviewed to determine whether an interview will be granted.

The Office of Admission encourages candidates who have been approved for an interview to request interviews in Grenada, and will schedule one upon the applicant's request. The University recognizes that financial considerations may prevent many candidates who reside at great distances from Grenada from choosing this option.

Interviews, therefore, may be conducted in the United States, the United Kingdom, Canada, the Caribbean, or other locations that best serve the diverse applicant pool. Candidates are advised that being granted an interview is no guarantee of acceptance; the interview itself plays a significant part in the decision by the Committee on Admission. Applicants are notified of the decision of the Committee on Admission. A record of the notification is kept for one year.

## ENTRANCE REQUIREMENTS

The requirements for direct entry into the four-year DVM program vary depending on the educational system of your home country. What is required for all applicants is completion of secondary school, a period of farm experience or time spent in a veterinary practice, and possession of a bachelors degree from an accredited University or 60 credit hours.

Specific undergraduate coursework (or its equivalent) is required as part of the preveterinary medical sciences requirements for admission.

Two letters of recommendation. In order of importance to the Committee on Admission, these are the categories:

a. A veterinarian with whom you have worked

b. A university professor (or, for those applying for the preveterinary program, a teacher)

c. A preveterinary advisor committee, or an advisor/counselor.

Two essays: A personal statement discussing the significant factors which led to your decision to pursue a career in veterinary medicine, and how you see yourself using this career to make a difference in the world (maximum 1500 words) and an additional essay explaining how you will contribute to the diversity of St. George's University (approximately 500 words).

*Applicants from North America*

A completed bachelors degree from an accredited university is required for direct entry into the four-year veterinary medical program. A candidate may apply before completion of the degree. Under exceptional circumstances a candidate may be considered with 60 undergraduate credit hours.

*Standardized Examination:* Candidates must submit scores by the corresponding application deadlines (see below) on the Graduate Record Examination or alternatively on the MCAT. (Our GRE Code is 7153; MCAT code 21303.)

*Applicants from Other Systems of Education*

For direct entry into the four-year DVM program, a bachelors degree with a strong science background is required.

Applicants with passes at the Advanced Level of the General Certificate of Education will be assessed individually and will be considered for appropriate entry into the five-year DVM program. Generally, A Level students with the appropriate courses and grades matriculate into the five-year veterinary medical program.

If English is not the principal language, the applicant must have achieved a score in the Test of English as a Foreign Language (TOEFL) of at least 600 points, 250 points computer-based or 100 points internet-based.

*Is a Bachelor's Degree Required?* yes

*Is this an International School?* yes

## ESTIMATED TUITION

*Estimated Tuition Resident:* $33,368

*Estimated Tuition Contract:* 0

*Estimated Tuition Non-Resident:* $33,368

## AVAILABLE SEATS

*Resident:* pending

*Contract:* 0

*Non-Resident:* pending

## TEST REQUIREMENTS

*Standardized Examination:* Candidates must submit scores by the corresponding application deadlines (see below) on the Graduate Record Examination or alternatively on the MCAT. (Our GRE Code is 7153; MCAT code 21303.)

*VMCAS Participation:* partial

*Accepts International Students?* yes

## ADDITIONAL INFORMATION

*Dual Degree Programs*

Combined DVM / MPH, MSc, and MBA degree programs are available. Applications can be submitted online directly through the SGU website at www.sgu.edu or via the VMCAS application system. If you have questions about the application process, please call one of our admission advisors at 1 (800) 899-6337, ext 9 1280.

*Application Deadline:* 10/2/2014

# UNIVERSITY OF SYDNEY

Faculty of Veterinary Science
JD Stewart building
University of Sydney
Sydney NSW 2006
Telephone: 02 9351 2441
Fax: 02 9351 3056
Email: vet.science@sydney.edu.au
Website: http://sydney.edu.au/vetscience

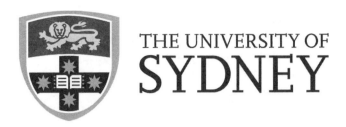

THE UNIVERSITY OF
## SYDNEY

## SCHOOL INFORMATION

The University of Sydney, founded in 1850, is Australia's first university. Over the past 150 years, the University has built an international reputation for its outstanding teaching and as a centre of research excellence. It is one of the largest universities in Australia, with over 47,000 students, including 9,000 international students from more than 100 different countries.

Located only ten minutes by bus from the heart of the Sydney business district, the main Camperdown campus provides easy access to Sydney's vibrant social scene, Sydney harbour and surrounds.

> The University of Sydney Faculty delivers inspirational and innovative student-centred teaching.

One of the best aspects of studying at the University of Sydney is that it is located in the most beautiful city in the 'down-under' country of Australia, and is a young, modern and bustling city that is very much alive.

The Faculty of Veterinary Science was established in 1910 and is the oldest continuing Faculty of its kind in Australia. The Faculty is an international leader in veterinary and animal education and is ranked 5/5 for Excellence in Research for Australia (ERA) for veterinary science research. The Faculty delivers inspirational and innovative student-centered teaching that leads to an acceptance of the need for life-long, evidence-based learning whilst also providing clinical and research excellence through creative, collaborative programs.

The exciting new Doctor of Veterinary Medicine (DVM) program aims to produce career ready graduates with excellent fundamental knowledge and skills in managing animal health and disease; and in protecting and advancing animal, human and environmental health and welfare locally and globally. Teaching is research-driven to so that students learn from the latest developments and advances in evidence-based practice, animal production, wildlife conservation, biomedical science, animal health, welfare and veterinary medicine, and veterinary public health in a global context. Clinical exposure, clinical skills training and animal handling commence in the first semester and continue throughout the course. The program culminates in a capstone experience year where students are placed as an intern in veterinary clinics of all varieties and in a wide range of locations, including rotations in the University teaching hospitals at Sydney and Camden.

The Faculty maintains teaching hospitals on both the inner-city Camperdown campus and the rural Camden campus, where students and veterinarians work together in a clinical teaching and learning environment. Referral and primary accession cases are seen at both sites. The University Veterinary Teaching Hospital at Camden also provides veterinary services to farms in the region., while the Wildlife Health and Conservation Clinic provides veterinary services to sick and injured Australian native wildlife, reptiles, avian, aquatic and exotic pets. A wide range of companion animals, farm animals, racing animals, exotic and native species are seen.

The DVM program produces graduates with the knowledge and skills to pursue many career options as veterinary scientists participating in the care and welfare of animals. Completion of the course ensures students have a wide knowledge of the principles associated with every aspect of health and disease in animals—domestic and native.

## ENTRY PATHWAYS

In 2015 the University of Sydney will have two pathways for students wishing to study veterinary medicine:

1. *Undergraduate applicants:* Students can apply for entry into a combined six-year Bachelor of Veterinary Biology/Doctor of Veterinary Medicine (BVetBiol/DVM) on the basis of their secondary school results (plus additional selection criteria). The BVetBiol/DVM commences with two years of undergraduate study in the Bachelor of Veterinary Biology and students who perform well will be eligible to progress to the Veterinary Medicine program in years 3-6.

2. *Graduate applicants:* Students may also complete a science-based bachelor degree from Sydney or any other institution and then apply for entry into the four-year DVM program.

Graduate students will need to have successfully completed at least one semester of study in general chemistry (physical and inorganic), organic chemistry, biology and biochemistry as part of their science degree.

## ADMISSION REQUIREMENTS

*Academic Performance:*

1. International students must have achieved a similar standard to that expected of an Australian student seeking entry.

   BVetBiol/DVM Undergraduate applicants will be assessed on the basis of their academic achievement in their final year of secondary education (Year 12 or equivalent) or their tertiary studies from a recognized University. Minimum GPA required for BVetBiol/DVM entry is 2.80 on a 4.00 scale, and applicants must demonstrate an aptitude for the sciences.

   DVM Graduate Applicants will be assessed on the basis of their completed Bachelor's degree from the University of Sydney or another institution. Minimum GPA required for DVM entry is 3.00 on a 4.00 scale. Graduates must have successfully completed the prerequisite subjects listed above.

2. *Standardized examinations (BVetBiol/DVM applicants only):* BVetBiol/DVM applicants must submit results from the International Student Admission Test (ISAT) http://www.acer.edu.au/isat. GRE scores may be submitted in lieu of ISAT scores. There is no standardized test for DVM Graduate entry

3. *Additional requirements and considerations:* All applicants are expected to have gained relevant work experience and animal handling. This should be demonstrated on the "Commitment to Veterinary Science" form that can be downloaded from the faculty web site http://sydney.edu.au/vetscience/future_students/

## PRACTICAL EXPERIENCE

During the inter-semester and intra-semester breaks students are required to undertake, placements for preparatory clinical and animal husbandry experience. The final year is lecture free with students participating in practice-based activities and the management and care of patients.

## PROFESSIONAL RECOGNITION

Sydney graduates are immediately eligible for registration for practice by all Australian state and territory veterinary surgeons' boards and are recognised by the Royal College of Veterinary Surgeons in the United Kingdom and the American Veterinary Medical Association.

## APPLICATION INFORMATION

All international applicants can apply directly to the University of Sydney using the on-line application system: http://sydney.edu.au/courses/

Prospective international students may obtain information about the University of Sydney from these University representatives: http://sydney.edu.au/future-students/international/undergraduate/find-an-agent.php

*Application deadline:* 31 October, however late applications will be considered if the quota has not been reached. Applications will be accepted throughout the year and assessed as soon as they are received.

For more information please visit the International Office website at http://sydney.edu.au/future-students

*Standardized test deadline for BVetBiol/DVM:* 31 October. Results must be submitted with application.

## NEW ENTRANTS

*Australian resident:* 90

*International:* 40

## TUITION FEES 2015 (INDICATIVE FEES)

*International student:* AUD$54,600

*Australian resident (government supported):* UD$10,388

*Australian resident:* AUD$48,000

Tuition fees are indexed annually.

# UTRECHT UNIVERSITY*

Office for International Cooperation
Faculty of Veterinary Medicine
Utrecht University
Yalelaan 1
3584 CL Utrecht
The Netherlands
Telephone: +31.30.2532116
Email: bic@vet.uu.nl
www.uu.nl/vet

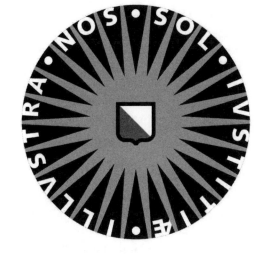

## SHORT HISTORY

In 1821 a state veterinary school was founded in Utrecht. Almost a century later, in 1918, the school acquired the status of an institution of higher learning and in 1925 it was incorporated into the State University of Utrecht and thereby became the first and until to date the only Faculty of Veterinary Medicine in the Netherlands. Utrecht University, founded in 1636, is one of the 14 universities in the Netherlands. The faculty of Veterinary Medicine is now one of the 6 faculties of Utrecht University and is located at campus site De Uithof just outside the city of Utrecht. The Faculty of Veterinary Medicine is housed in modern and spacious buildings on a total surface of 60.000 m.

> Utrecht University, is one of the 14 universities in the Netherlands and is located at campus site De Uithof.

## ORGANISATION AND STAFF

The faculty encompasses 8 departments with specialized facilities, a Faculty Office and a number of general services (e.g. leaning environment with audio- visual units and the library, pharmacy, experimental farms, museum, student computer rooms etc). The faculty has an academic staff of 418 fte, including 32 full professors and an administrative and support staff of 484 fte. Most staff members can communicate well in English and most lecturers have experience in teaching veterinary medicine in the English language.

## VETERINARY EDUCATION

Admission of students to the 6-year veterinary training programme (taught in Dutch) is limited to 225 each year, resulting in a total of 1400 students. The veterinary curriculum leads to the "dierenarts' degree (Doctor of Veterinary Medicine, DVM). In September 2007 the veterinary education under a Bachelor - Master (3+3 years) structure started with the 1st year of the bachelor programme.

## RESEARCH AND POSTGRADUATE EDUCATION

Research at the faculty of Veterinary Medicine is the responsibility of the Institute for Veterinary Research (IVR). Research which is conducted as part of the postgraduate master programmes and PhD programme is linked to one of the research programmes of the IVR. The postgraduate master programmes were initiated from 1994 onwards and are now integrated in the postgraduate educational Master of Science programme Veterinary Science.

## QUALITY OF EDUCATION

The faculty of Veterinary Medicine is accredited by the American Veterinary Medical Association (AVMA) and Canadian Veterinary Medical Association (CVMA) since 1973, the European Association of Establishments of Veteri- nary Education and the Dutch and Flemish Accreditation Organization.

*These pages are for last year's admissions cycle. For updated information, please visit: http://www.uu.nl/university/international-students/EN/admission/Pages/default.aspx

## INFORMATION ABOUT THE ADMISSION TO THE FACULTY OF VETERINARY MEDICINE FOR FOREIGN STUDENTS

Special rules apply for the study of Veterinary Medicine. The Dutch Ministry of Education has declared the so-called numerus fixus applicable to the study of Veterinary Medicine. This entails that only a limited amount of students is admitted each year. The number of admission requests largely exceeds the number of allocations. Those restrictions affect both Dutch and foreign students. The available places are assigned by selection through interviews or drawing lots.

### APPLICATION AND DRAWING LOTS

Each year the minister of Education and Science determines the number of students that can be admitted to the study of Veterinary Medicine. At this moment the number is 225. In order to take part in the lottery for placement, you need to complete an application form via Internet (start with website: www. uu.nl) and send this in <u>before May 15th</u>.

If you do not apply you cannot participate in drawing lots.

### FOREIGN DIPLOMAS

Foreign diplomas have to be evaluated and compared with the Dutch equivalent diplomas. This evaluation takes time and can result in the fact that you have to take supplementary exams before being accepted for the lottery.

Information about the evaluation of your diplomas can be obtained at:

Universiteit Utrecht, Admissions Office
P.O. Box 80 125, 3508 TC Utrecht, the Netherlands
Phone: +31 30 253 7000
Visiting Address: Leuvenlaan 19, Utrecht – De Uithof

### DUTCH LANGUAGE EXAM

If the result of the lottery is favorable, then - prior to admission to the study of Veterinary Medicine - you have to prove your (sufficient) knowledge of the Dutch language. This is a requirement under the Dutch law because the education is in the Dutch language. The owner of a foreign diploma therefore has to pass the exam "Dutch as Second Language program 2" (*Staatsexamen Nederlands als Tweede Taal, programma 2*) before being admitted.

Request information about language courses and the examinations at:

James Boswell Institute
P.O. Box 80148, 3508 TC Utrecht, The Netherlands
Phone: +31 30 253 8666

## TUITION FEES AND SCHOLARSHIPS

The tuition fee depends on your nationality and the programme you register for:

*Tuition 2012-2013*

EU / EEA: Bachelor's and Master's programmes: €1,771

Non EU / EEA: Bachelor Veterinary Medicine: €10,500

Non EU / EEA: Master Veterinary Medicine: €19,500

No financial aid is offered to foreign students. Neither the government nor the university grants scholarships to foreign students.

### RESIDENCE PERMIT

Every foreign student who wants to receive academic education in the Netherlands needs a residence permit. More information can be obtained at the Admissions Office.

### DOCUMENTATION

When requesting admission, the following pieces of documentation have to be sent to the Admissions Office (see above):

- a short and concise curriculum vitae with a complete overview of the education

- a certified copy of the birth register

- certified copies of diplomas, subject overview, list of marks of secondary and (pre-) university education in Dutch, French, German, or English

- a copy of personal details from the passport

For further information about the admission to the study of Veterinary Medicine please contact:

Student advisor
Faculty of Veterinary Medicine
Department of Educational and Student Affairs/Office for International Cooperation
PO Box 80 163, 3508 TD Utrecht, the Netherlands
e-mail: osz@vet.uu.nl

# UNIVERSITY OF COPENHAGEN

Office for International Cooperation
Faculty of Health and Medical Sciences
University of Copenhagen
Blegdamsvej 3B
DK-2200 København N
Denmark
Telephone: +45 35 33 35 89
Email: hhd@sund.ku.dk
www.sund.ku.dk

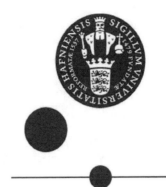

UNIVERSITY OF
COPENHAGEN

## ST. SHORT HISTORY

The Veterinary School in Copenhagen was founded in 1773 as one of the first schools in the world. In 1856 the veterinary school was moved to its present location and at that time acquired the status of an institution of higher learning incorporating agriculture and animal science. In 2007 the Royal Veterinary and Agricultural University merged with the University of Copenhagen and was transformed into the Faculty of Life Sciences incorporating the veterinary school. The University of Copenhagen was inaugurated on 1 June 1479, after King Christian I was granted approval for its establishment by Pope Sixtus IV. Based on a German model, the university consisted of four faculties: Theology, Law, Medicine and Philosophy. Today with more than 38,000 students and more than 9,000 employees, the University of Copenhagen is the largest institution of research and education in Denmark. The purpose of the University – to quote the University Statute – is to 'conduct research and provide further education to the highest academic level'.

> The University of Copenhagen is the largest institution of research and education in Denmark.

Approximately one hundred different institutes, departments, laboratories, centers, museums, etc., form the nucleus of the University, where professors, lecturers and other academic staff, as well as most of the technical and administrative personnel, carry out their daily work, and where teaching takes place. With the opening of the totally rebuilt and modernized Small Animal University Hospital at the Frederiksberg Campus in early 2011 the Copenhagen Veterinary School including the newly built Large Animal University Hospital at the Taastrup Campus functions as one of the most modern veterinary schools with state of the art equipment.

In 2012 the Copenhagen School of Veterinary Medicine together with the School of Pharmaceutical Sciences merged with the Faculty of Health to form a new, scientifically and financially strong Faculty of Health and Medicine within the University of Copenhagen.

## ORGANIZATION AND STAFF

The veterinary school encompasses 3 departments with specialized facilities, a Faculty Office and a number of general services (e.g. learning environment with audio-visual units, library, , experimental farms, student facilities including several computer rooms etc). The veterinary school has an academic staff of 154 fte, including 29 full professors and an administrative and support staff of 221 fte. Most staff members communicate well in English and all academic staff members have experience in teaching veterinary medicine in English. In early 2012 all academic staff members have completed officially approved proficiency tests in English.

## UNDERGRADUATE VETERINARY EDUCATION

Admission of students to the 5½-year undergraduate veterinary training program is limited to 180 each year, resulting in a total of 1100 students. They pass full examinations at the completion of each course.

## RESEARCH AND POSTGRADUATE EDUCATION

Research at the School of Veterinary Medicine is the responsibility of the Vice Dean for Research and the department heads. Research which is conducted as part of the PhD programs is included in this portfolio.

## QUALITY OF EDUCATION

The School of Veterinary Medicine, Faculty of Health and Medicine within the University of Copenhagen has been regularly evaluated and accredited by the European Association of Establishments of Veterinary Education since 1988 (latest accreditation in 2010) and had a pre-site Visit by the American Veterinary Medical Association (AVMA) in 2009. A full AVMA site visit is scheduled for April 2015.

## INFORMATION ABOUT THE ADMISSION TO THE FACULTY OF VETERINARY MEDICINE FOR FOREIGN STUDENTS

In general foreign students have access to the Danish universities. Non-EU citizens must apply for visa before being allowed to apply.

Special rules apply for the study of Veterinary Medicine. The Danish Ministry of Science has declared a numerous clauses to the DVM program. This entails that only a limited amount of students is admitted each year. The number of admission requests largely exceeds the number of allocations. Restrictions affect both Danish and foreign students. The available places are assigned by selection through interviews (50%) or based upon grades obtained in high school (50%). Letters of recommendation are neither required nor accepted.

## APPLICATION TO THE DANISH DVM PROGRAM

Each year the minister of education and science lays down the number of students to be admitted to the DVM program. Currently 180 students are accepted in each class. There are two routes of application. The first is solely based upon high school grades (Quota I) and the second is based upon a mixture of high school grades, working experience and an interview (Quota II). No standardized tests are required before application. Application deadline for Quota I is 5 July 2014, and for Quota II the application deadline is 15 March 2014.

International students are referred to http://studier.ku.dk/internationalstudents/ for further information about application for the Danish DVM program.

## TUITION FEES AND SCHOLARSHIPS

Generally students from within the European Union do not pay tuition fee. For foreign students please refer to web site of the Ministry of Science, Technology and Innovation http://en.vtu.dk/ . Generally financial aid is not offered to foreign students.

## RESIDENCE PERMIT

Foreign students who want to receive an academic education in Denmark need a residence permit. More information can be obtained at the Office for International Cooperation or at a Danish embassy in the country of origin.

Additionally applicants must demonstrate access to sufficient financial means. The amount varies and more detailed information should be sought at a Danish embassy.

# ST. MATTHEWS UNIVERSITY

Email Address: admissions@stmatthews.edu
Website: www.stmatthews .edu

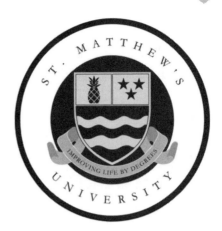

## SCHOOL DESCRIPTION

St. Matthew's University School of Veterinary Medicine is located on beautiful Grand Cayman in the Caribbean. Grand Cayman is the fifth largest financial district in the world and has a highly developed infrastructure which is very com parable to the United States. It is also one of the safest islands in the Caribbean, boasting one of the lowest crime and poverty rates. Grand Cayman has hundreds of restaurants, scores of banks, world-class hotels, and many opportunities for boating, diving, horseback riding, and other recreation. The island is less than an hours flight from Miami, and also has direct flights from Atlanta, Chicago, Charlotte, Houston, Tampa, Toronto, Washington D.C., and other locations.

> Throughout your ten semesters at St. Matthew's University, we will support all aspects of your education and life.

At SMU, we are as committed to your dreams as you are. Throughout your ten semesters with us, we will do everything we can to ensure your success by supporting all aspects of your education and life, including:

*Focus on Teaching:* Dedicated, talented faculty whose time commitments are focused on reaching and mentoring.

*Student Mentors:* Student mentors understand about adjusting to life in veterinary school, and are eager to see you succeed.

*Very Low Student to Faculty Ratio:* With a student to faculty ratio of less than five to one, you will have an unprecedented level of faculty support and attention.

We limit each incoming cohort of students to a maximum of 30.

*Best Value:* Most affordable tuition of any Caribbean veterinary school. Accelerated Schedule: Complete your pre-clinical education on Grand Cayman in just 28 months, and then return to the U.S. or Canada for clinical training, with the ability to complete vet school in just over three years.

SMU's modern, state-of-the-art main campus is located across the street from beautiful Seven Mile Beach, and boasts wireless technology throughout the bright, air-conditioned classrooms, labs, library, and student lounges. SMU also has a Clinical Teaching Facility which hosts surgery, medicine and clinical skills training as well as anatomy and pathology laboratories. Students have the opportunity to travel to local farms with veterinary staff from the Cayman Department of Agriculture. Our students spend seven (7) semesters on Grand Cayman and their final months in clinical programs at one of our many AVMA-accredited Clinical Program Affiliate Schools in the United States and Canada.

There arc significant opportunities for students to gain experience with exotic species through our collaborations with the Cayman Turtle Farm, Central Caribbean Marine Institute, Dolphin Discovery, the Blue Iguana Project and the Marine Research Program.

## APPLICATION INFORMATION

We welcome applications from any qualified candidate who dreams of become a veterinarian. For specific application information (availability, deadlines, feeds, transferring to SMU and VMCAS participation), please refer to the contact information above.

## SUMMARY OF ADMISSIONS PROCEDURES

*Timetable:*

*Application deadlines:* none. Rolling admissions. Three incoming cohorts per year.

*Interviews:* Held in person or via telephone/videoconference.

*School begins:* August, January, May (three start dates per year).

*Deposit (to hold a place in class):* $500.00

*Deferments:* Considered on an individual basis.

Transfer applications for admission with advanced standings are welcome. Transfer credits (advance standing) may be awarded at the discretion of the University. No transfers are permitted after than beginning of Semester 5.

*Seats generally available:* Maximum of 30 (total) seats available per incoming cohort to ensure exceptional level of faculty support for students.

## ENTRANCE REQUIREMENTS

All prerequisite courses must be completed prior to matriculation.

*Is a Bachelor's Degree Required?* no

*Is this an International School?* yes

## ESTIMATED TUITION

*Estimated Tuition Resident:* Pre-Clinical Sciences (Grand Cayman): $11,375

*Estimated Tuition Contract:* Clinical Sciences (Clinical Affiliates): $18,500

*Estimated Tuition Non-Resident:* Additional Fees: $2,755

## AVAILABLE SEATS

*Resident:* 0

*Contract:* 0

*Non-Resident:* 30

## TEST REQUIREMENTS

Graduate Record Examination (GRE), general test, is not required but is recommended.

*VMCAS Participation:* non-VMCAS

*Accepts International Students?* yes

## ADDITIONAL INFORMATION

The admissions team at SMU wants to get to know you! To us, you are much more than a GPA or GRE score. We want to know about you as a person because ultimately, that is what will determine the kind of veterinarian you will be. We want to support you in your dram of becoming a veterinarian, and we welcome your application!

*Application Deadline:* rolling

# UNIVERSITY OF TOKYO

Graduate School of Agricultural and Life Sciences
The University of Tokyo
1-1-1, Yayoi, Bunkyo-ku, Tokyo, 113-8657

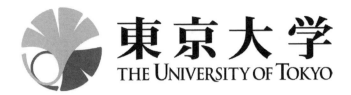

東京大学
THE UNIVERSITY OF TOKYO

## SCHOOL DESCRIPTION

Veterinary medicine covers wide areas of life sciences, not only medicine for animals but also biology of mammals and higher vertebrates. In the Department of Veterinary Medicine, most advanced research is being carried out at molecular, cellular and in vivo levels, in order to fully understand vital processes of normal and diseased animals. Veterinary medicine has two aspects of science: basic science to understand the mechanisms underlying biological phenomena, and applied science to satisfy the social demands for maintenance and improvement of human welfare and productivity of domestic animals. This department collaborates with the veterinary medical center located on the Yayoi campus. This center is facilitated with the latest and most advanced medical instruments, and plays an important role as an advanced veterinary hospital in this area.

> The Department of Veterinary Medicine collaborates with the veterinary medical center located on the Yayoi campus.

## FOR MORE INFORMATION

For more information about the University of Tokyo's Veterinary Medicine Program, please go to the following website: http://www.u-tokyo.ac.jp/en/admissions-and-programs/graduate-and-research/graduate-schools/agricultural.html

# UNIVERSIDAD VERITAS

Escuela de Medicina y Cirugía Veterinaria
San Francisco de Asís
San Rafael de Coronado
Tel: (506) 2292-7639
Tel: (506) 2292-6811
Tel: (506) 2294-3292
E-mail: info@veterinariaveritas.ac.cr

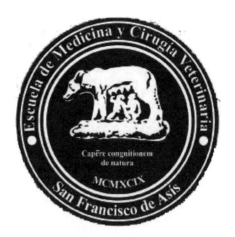

## PROCESS OF ADMISSION AND REGISTRATION

*1. Admission Process*

Return ANNEX 2 completely filled out with the following documentation:

a. Handwritten Application. Write why would you like to study veterinary medicine (a few sentences).
b. Original and photocopy of your high school diploma.
c. Two recent color photos, passport size.
d. For Costa Rican adults: a photocopy of your "Cédula." For minors: a photocopy of both sides the "Cédula de Menores."
e. Grades from your senior year in high school.
f. For foreigners: a photocopy of your current passport and a notarized copy of your high school diploma by the Embassy of Costa Rica in your home country, attaching the Apostille Convention certificate to be properly validated by the Departamento de Control de Calidad (Quality Control Dept.) by the Ministerio de Educación in Costa Rica.
g. All documents must be translated in Spanish by the Ministry of Foreign Affairs.

> Located in San Rafael de Coronado in Costa Rica, the Universidad Veritas is an affiliate member of the AAVMC.

*2. Registration Process*

a. December, April, and August, to submit the completed form.
b. Registration will be held on the third week of the months mentioned above.
c. Enrollment schedule 8:00 AM, 11:30 AM, 1:30 PM, to 4:00 PM.
d. Classes begin first day of January, May, and September of each year.

In the first level, Training Seminar I (uvmv015) is mandatory; therefore, the student must enroll in this subject.

Note: For the second period of 2014, the quota for new students is 50.

The admitted students will be contacted.

*3. Payment*

a. For cash registration and tuition payment, on enrollment day you must bring the deposit receipt issued by a bank. Foreigners pay in US dollars.
b. There is a possibility to be funded by CONAPE. Students must bring canceled registration and poof of CONAPE's loan approval.
c. Line of credit (just for citizen): those interested should ask at Reception for a credit form and return it on enrollment day. You must cancel registration and the third part of tuition, and bring your canceled receipt.
d. Card payment.

# POLICIES ON ADVANCED STANDING

Transfers are permitted to most colleges of veterinary medicine in the United States under specified conditions. Typical requirements include a vacancy in the class, completion of all prerequisite requirements, and compatible curricula. Following is a listing of schools and some of the conditions under which they will consider a transfer from another veterinary college with advanced standing. More detailed information may be obtained by writing to the individual schools in which you have an interest.

## UNITED STATES

### UNIVERSITY OF CALIFORNIA, DAVIS

Applications may be considered if available positions exist within the third-year classes. Currently, each class in the DVM program of the School of Veterinary Medicine shall consist of no more than 138 students.

1. The applicant must have a strong academic record in his/her undergraduate program.
2. The applicant must be currently enrolled in an AVMA-accredited DVM program and must be in excellent academic and ethical standing in that program. The specific minimum benchmark will be that the applicant is in the top quartile of students in the Veterinary School in which the applicant is currently enrolled as determined by GPA or class rank.
3. The applicant must have completed veterinary course work equivalent to that expected of the students in the DVM program of the School of Veterinary Medicine, UC Davis, who will be in the same academic class.
4. The applicant has a valid reason for requesting admission in advanced standing.

### UNIVERSITY OF FLORIDA

1. An opening must exist in the second- or third-year class.
2. Students are only rarely considered for advanced standing based on exceptional personal circumstances.
3. Student must be enrolled in an AVMA accredited college.
4. Student must meet all prerequisites for admission as a first-year student (including GRE® scores).
5. The curricula of the two schools must be sufficiently alike to allow a student to enter without deficiencies in academic background.

6. Applicants must have a letter approving transfer from their dean or associate dean.

### University of Georgia

1. Priority is given to Georgia residents, followed by contract state residents, then all other applicants.
2. Applicants will be considered for entry into the DVM degree program up to the third year of the curriculum, when and if space is available, as defined by the Admissions Committee.
3. Applications must include official transcripts of all completed veterinary and pre-veterinary coursework and a letter of support written by a senior administrator of the school in which the applicant is currently enrolled stating the applicant is currently in good academic standing.
4. No individual is eligible for transfer who has been dismissed or is on probation at any other school or college for deficiency in scholarship or because of misconduct.

### UNIVERSITY OF ILLINOIS

1. Transfer students will only be considered for the beginning of the second year of veterinary medicine and only if transfer seats become available in that class.
2. All prerequisite science courses must be completed prior to the request for transfer.
3. Minimum grade requirements include:
   cumulative and science GPAs of 2.75 on a 4.00 scale (doesn't include veterinary work); results of the Graduate Record Examination General Test completed within the last two years.
4. Student must complete the same preveterinary coursework as required for students accepted to the first year of the program.
5. Student must be in good academic standing.
6. To be considered for transfer, a student must present credentials for preprofessional work that fulfill the University of Illinois College of Veterinary Medicine requirements for first-year entry.
7. Complete information and an application can be found at vetmed.illinois.edu/asa/brochure.

### COLORADO STATE UNIVERSITY

Transfer is dependent on position openings in the year into which the student transfers (most transfers will involve the loss of a year because of differences in school curricula). Candidate must:

1. have successfully completed at least the first year (equivalent of two semesters) of veterinary curriculum at an AVMA accredited college of veterinary medicine.

AND

2. have obtained the equivalent of a 3.0 cumulative GPA in your veterinary program AND must not have received a D, F, or unsatisfactory grade of any kind since enrolling in veterinary school.

AND

3. have a preveterinary academic record comparable to currently enrolled DVM students.

AND

4. provide evidence of noncognitive attributes comparable to currently enrolled DVM students.

If a veterinary student with an interest in transferring to CSU's DVM program meets ALL of the above minimum requirements, he/she may apply to the DVM program. To apply for transfer to CSU's Veterinary Program, please see http://www.cvmbs.colostate.edu/ns/_docs/students/dvm_policy_transfer_students.pdf.

## CORNELL UNIVERSITY

1. Students are considered for advanced standing in rare and exceptional circumstances. Each request for transfer is considered on an individual basis.

2. Transfer students will be considered if an opening exists in the second-year class. Students seeking advanced standing may enter the DVM program at two points: at the beginning of the second year of study, or mid-way through the second year, at the beginning of the fourth (Spring) semester of study.

3. Students seeking advanced standing must be enrolled in an AVMA-accredited veterinary college.

4. The curricula of the two schools must be sufficiently similar to allow students to enter without deficiencies in their academic background.

5. Students must meet all pre-veterinary requirements for first-year entry at the College of Veterinary Medicine at Cornell University (including GRE scores, prerequisite coursework, animal and veterinary experience), and may not have any failing grades on their veterinary transcript.

6. Scores from the Graduate Record Examination (GRE) or Medical College Admissions Test (MCAT) may not be older than five years.

7. Applicants seeking advanced standing must include a letter from their Associate Dean certifying that the student is in good academic standing, has not been on academic probation, and has not been subject to any disciplinary action or dismissal for any reason.

8. Applicants are required to have completed at least two full semesters at the institution from which the transfer is requested. Only veterinary coursework completed at an AVMA-accredited institution will be considered.

9. After analyzing the academic background of the applicant, the Admissions Committee will place each accepted transfer student in the semester of study in the DVM curriculum deemed most appropriate. (Veterinary course syllabi will be required at time of application).

## IOWA STATE UNIVERSITY

Acceptance of students for advanced standing is on the recommendation of the Academic Standards Committee. Space must be available in the class to which the student is applying. See website, http://vetmed.iastate.edu/academics/prospective-students/admissions/transfer-admissions, for the transfer application form and further details.

## KANSAS STATE UNIVERSITY

Acceptance of students for transfer is on recommendation of the Admissions Committee on a space-available basis.

## LOUISIANA STATE UNIVERSITY

1. There must be a vacancy in the class.

2. The curricula must be compatible.

3. The student must be in good academic standing with at least a 3.2 GPA in veterinary coursework at his/her present college.

4. Admission is limited to the second year of the program and only into the fall semester.

5. Each request for transfer is considered on a case-by-case basis.

6. To initiate the transfer process, please carefully read the DVM Transfer Guidelines information at www.vetmed.lsu.edu/admissions/transferapps.asp.

## MICHIGAN STATE UNIVERSITY

1. Admission consideration is offered only to those current matriculants in professional veterinary curricula who believe that there are extenuating circumstances that would precipitate significant undue hardship if they continue at their current institution.

2. Applicants requesting a transfer must contact the Dean of Academic and Student Affairs at the school they are currently attending and notify him or her of their intent.

3. Applicants must also demonstrate quality academic performance throughout their professional school enrollment.
4. The curricula of the two schools must be sufficiently alike to allow a student to enter the second-year class without deficiencies in academic background.
5. All selection criteria for regular applicants apply to transfer applicants.
6. Priority is given to Michigan residents.
7. Applicants who have previously been denied admission to MSU CVM will not be considered for transfer admissions.
8. Space must be available.
9. AVMA accreditation of current school is considered.

## UNIVERSITY OF MINNESOTA

1. Transfer students are accepted on a space available basis. The Admissions Committee will place each applicant in the year or semester of the curriculum deemed appropriate after analysis of equivalency of the required courses involved.
2. No academic work or standing will be accepted from DVM curricula other than those deemed accredited by the American Veterinary Medical Association.
3. All applicants must be U.S. citizens or holders of appropriate visas.
4. All applicants are required to have finished at least one full academic year at the institution from which transfer is requested and must be in good academic standing at the time of discontinuance according to written verification from the institution.
5. All applicants must have achieved a cumulative GPA of 3.00 (of 4.00) for the required courses at the initial institution.
6. Please visit the following website for more details: http://www.cvm.umn.edu/education/prospective/transferring/home.html

## MISSISSIPPI STATE UNIVERSITY

The Mississippi State University College of Veterinary Medicine accepts, on a limited basis, transfer students from other veterinary medical colleges to fill vacancies in the freshmen or sophomore classes. Transfer guidelines are as follows:

*From a veterinary school not accredited by the AVMA:*

Applicants for transfer into the second semester of the first year must have completed coursework equivalent to coursework taught in the first semester of the first year at MSU-CVM.

Applicants for transfer into the first semester of the second year must have completed coursework equivalent to coursework taught in the first year at MSU-CVM.

Applicants for transfer into the second semester of the second year must have completed coursework equivalent to all coursework taught in the first three semesters at MSU-CVM plus have had equivalent surgery laboratories.

*From a veterinary school accredited by the AVMA:*

Applicants are considered on a case-by-case basis with regard to length of time in current program.

*General:*

Any applicant considered for transfer admission must be in good academic standing (defined as being eligible to continue at current school from current point in the curriculum), never have failed a course while in veterinary medical school, never have been dismissed from a veterinary school and must have completed at least a full academic year at current veterinary school.

Any applicants considered for transfer admission will be required to attend an interview at Mississippi State University.

Typically, transfer applicants are not accepted into our program at a point later than first semester of the sophomore year. Accordingly, if a student should pursue application to Mississippi State University College of Veterinary Medicine and be accepted, it would be necessary for that student to complete at least two years at Mississippi State University to be eligible for a degree.

Students accepted for transfer are required to meet the current computer requirements of the college.

For more information, contact Tonya Calmes, Admissions Assistant, 662-325-4161, tcalmes@cvm.msstate.edu.

## UNIVERSITY OF MISSOURI

1. Must be a vacancy in the class.
2. Will consider students who are U.S. citizens or holders of permanent alien visas and who have finished at least two years in a college of veterinary medicine that is AVMA accredited.
3. Students must be in good academic standing, never been denied admission from the University of Missouri for a first year position, and submit a letter of reference from the dean's office of the present college is required.

## NORTH CAROLINA STATE UNIVERSITY

1. Must be a vacancy in the class.
2. Consideration by the Admission Committee on an individual basis.

3. Curricula must be compatible.
4. A letter from the dean of the current school certifying the applicant's academic standing.
5. Letter of recommendation from a faculty member at the original college.
6. Only accept transfers from AVMA accredited colleges.
7. At least 50% of DVM credit hours must be completed at North Carolina State in order to earn a North Carolina State University degree.

## THE OHIO STATE UNIVERSITY

The Ohio State University does not accept transfer students.

## OKLAHOMA STATE UNIVERSITY

Transfer students are considered. Each application is evaluated on an individual basis. See website for transfer guide. http://www.cvhs.okstate.edu

## OREGON STATE UNIVERSITY

Admission of students with advanced standing is considered only in certain circumstances, and each case is considered on an individual basis.

## UNIVERSITY OF PENNSYLVANIA

PennVet does not consider transfer applications.

## PURDUE UNIVERSITY

1. Positions must be available in the relevant class.
2. Student must be in good academic standing in his/her present program.
3. Students must have completed 1–2 years of DVM courses with an **exceptional** academic record in those courses.
4. Veterinary medical curricula must be compatible.
5. Student must have support of the administration from the program in which he/she is currently enrolled.

Please visit the following website for more specific detail: http://www.vet.purdue.edu/dvm/files/documents/transfer_policy.pdf

## UNIVERSITY OF TENNESSEE

Admission of students with advanced standing (transfer) may be considered for unique circumstances on a case-by-case basis.

1. Position(s) must be available in the class into which one would like to matriculate.
2. Curricula of the two schools must be sufficiently alike to allow a student to matriculate without deficiencies in his/her academic background.

3. The applicant's academic dean must provide a letter approving transfer and indicating that the student is in good standing at his/her current college/school of veterinary medicine.
4. Admission is usually limited to the second semester of the first year of the DVM curriculum except for exceptional circumstances.
5. Letters of reference are required.

The Admissions Committee will review applicant credentials and interview those determined to best meet admission criteria.

## TEXAS A & M UNIVERSITY

Students requesting advanced standing must meet the following requirements:

1. Must have completed all previous professional veterinary courses in an AVMA accredited college of veterinary medicine.
2. Must have successfully completed the academic term preceding the semester into which student requests admission.
3. Must comply with all requirements for transfer into the university as described in the current catalog.
4. May request transfer only into the second through seventh semesters of the professional curriculum.
5. At the time of matriculation the student must certify by letter that he/she has not been convicted of crimes in the period from first enrollment in the college of veterinary medicine from which the student desires transfer until date of matriculation at Texas A&M University.
6. To request transfer consideration, the student must meet all requirements as posted on the College website at http://www.cvm.tamu.edu/dcvm/admissions/transferpol.shtml.

## TUFTS UNIVERSITY

Applicants from other veterinary schools are considered. Students with advanced standing are admitted if and when space becomes available in the second-year class. The application deadline is June 1 for the following September. Please refer to our web site for details: http://www.tufts.edu/vet/

## TUSKEGEE UNIVERSITY

*General:* In most instances, transfer of a DVM student from their current program into the DVM program at Tuskegee will not be possible. However, in some cases transfer can be accomplished if a series of criteria can be met.

*Criteria required for transfer:* There are six specific criteria that must be met in order for a DVM student matriculating at another veterinary school or college of veterinary medicine to transfer into the DVM program at Tuskegee University School of Veterinary Medicine (TUSVM). These criteria are listed below.

1. The student seeking transfer to TUSVM must be currently enrolled in a school or college of veterinary medicine that is fully accredited by the American Veterinary Medical Association Counsel ob Education,

2. The student seeking to transfer to TUSVM must be in good academic standing at the veterinary school or college they are matriculating.

3. The DVM curriculum at the perspective transferees' school or college of matriculation must be sufficiently similar to the DVM curriculum at TUSVM to make transfer possible.

4. The perspective transferees' reason(s) for wanting to effect a transfer from their current DVM program to the DVM program at TUSVM must be evaluated and deemed an appropriate reason(s).

5. The perspective transferee must have either the Associate Dean For Academic Affairs or the Dean of their current DVM program submit a letter to the Director of Veterinary Admissions at TUSVM which specifically reaffirms the reason(s) for wanting to transfer and which also states that the perspective transferee is not under any present non-academic probationary status or under any present or pending disciplinary action(s).

6. The transfer must be approved by the Dean of the Tuskegee University College of Veterinary Medicine, Nursing, and Allied Health.

## VIRGINIA-MARYLAND REGIONAL COLLEGE OF VETERINARY MEDICINE

VMRCVM accepts students for advanced standing on the recommendation of the Admissions Committee on a space-available basis.

## WASHINGTON STATE UNIVERSITY

Admission of students with advanced standing is considered only in very specific and unique circumstances, and each case is considered on an individual basis.

## UNIVERSITY OF WISCONSIN

Wisconsin does not accept advanced standing students for admission.

## INTERNATIONAL

## MASSEY UNIVERSITY

Applications for admission with advanced standing will only be considered by students enrolled in a veterinary program with a compatible curriculum, and pending an available space in the appropriate stage of the program. Applicants should contact vetschool@massey.ac.nz to apply for advanced standing.

## MURDOCH UNIVERSITY

Applications for advanced standing will only be considered from students whose studies have been completed in a DVM program. Applicants are required to apply formally for advanced standing and provide the necessary documentation to allow for a full comparison between the previous study and Murdoch University's unit requirements. Prior courses must duplicate or substantially overlap multiple factors including breadth and depth of content, duration, objectives, assessment, context, and academic standard (level of intellectual effort required) for exemption to be granted.

## ST. MATTHEW'S UNIVERSITY

Applications for admission with advanced standing are welcomed from students from veterinary schools recognized by the American Veterinary Medical Association (AVMA) and/or the American Association of Veterinary State Boards (AAVSB). Transfer applicants must submit a complete application package to ensure a timely review. Acceptance of transfer credit is at the discretion of St. Matthew's University.

## UNIVERSITY OF CALGARY

Applications for admission to advanced semesters may be considered from students who have been enrolled in DVM programs at other institutions, subject to the availability of spaces in the DVM Program and the academic standing of the candidate. When places are available, candidates may be asked to present themselves for an interview and may be asked to pass examinations on subject matter in the veterinary curriculum. Applicants are advised that vacancies are rare and that restrictions on residency and citizenship status may be applied.

## UNIVERSITY OF PRINCE EDWARD ISLAND

Applicants who have completed all or portions of a veterinary medical program may apply for advanced standing to the second year of the DVM program.

Applicants for advanced standing must present evidence of educational accomplishments and may be required to address missing courses or competencies expected of our incoming second-year students. Students admitted with advanced standing must begin the college year in September.

The candidate must file a formal application and may be interviewed by the Admissions Committee and possibly other faculty. Places for admission to the college with advanced standing are limited and depend on vacancies.

It is imperative that the Admissions Committee have detailed and translated summaries of veterinary medical academic programs and accomplishments for those seeking advanced placement from schools in foreign countries.

Advanced-standing applications should be on file and completed as early as possible and no later than January 1. Candidates are strongly encouraged to visit the website http://www.upei.ca/programsandcourses/transfer-and-advanced-standing-applicants-dvm.

## UNIVERSITY OF QUEENSLAND

Applications for advanced standing will only be considered from students whose studies have been completed in a veterinary program with a compatible curriculum, and where a space is available in the appropriate stage of the program. Please refer to the University of Queensland Policy 3.50.03 - Credit for Previous Studies and Recognised Prior Learning (http://ppl.app.uq.edu.au/) or contact the School directly (vetenquiries@uq.edu.au).

## UNIVERSITY OF SASKATCHEWAN

Applications for admission with advanced standing will only be considered if a vacancy in the Year II class develops. Students applying for advanced standing must meet the normal residency requirements and must be enrolled in a program that has a compatible curriculum. Applicants are required to complete a formal application form and, dependent on their academic record, will be considered for an interview. Part of the interview will be an assessment of their current knowledge. If English is not their first language, applicants will also be required to submit a TOEFL score. Admission is not considered beyond the second year of the program.

# Enrolled First-Year Students by State*Residency at the Time of Application

American Students Only
AAVMC Internal Reports
2014

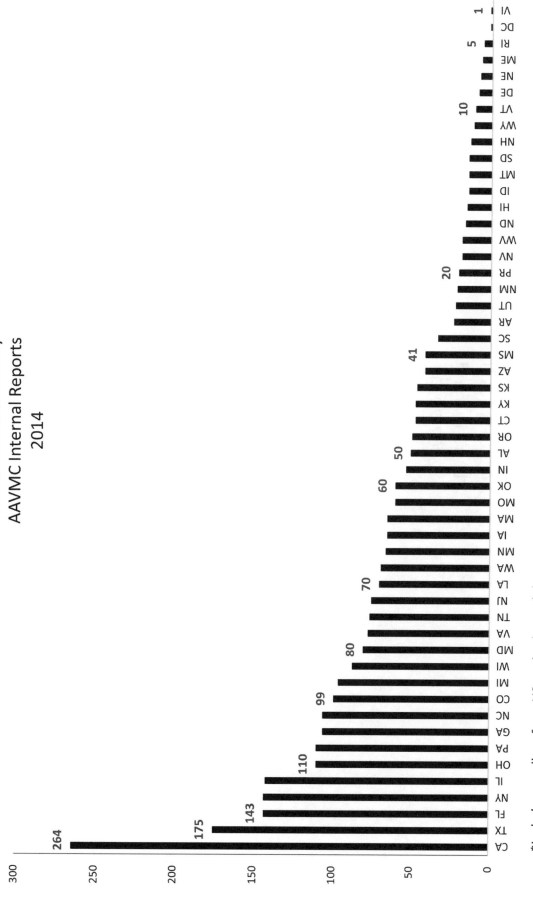

*Includes enrollees from US territories and the District of Columbia

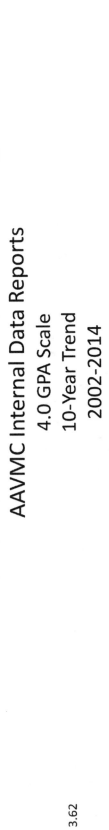
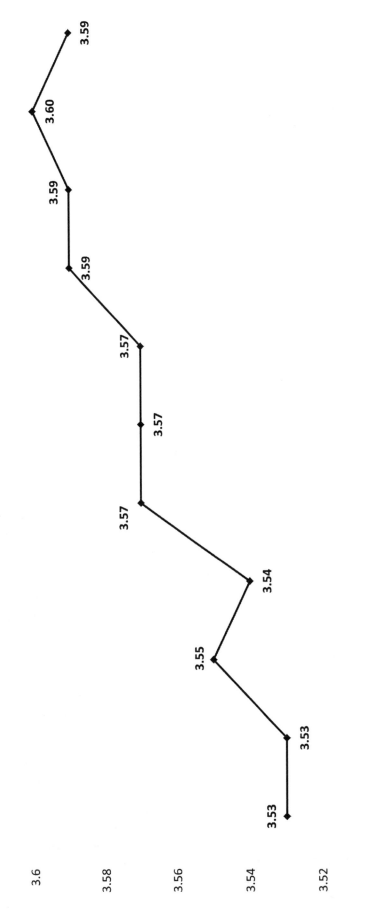

# First-Year Student Pre-Vet Grade Point Average

AAVMC Internal Data Reports

4.0 GPA Scale
10-Year Trend
2002-2014

# Veterinary College Applicants and Available First-Year Positions

## VMCAS Participating Institutions Only*

### AAVMC Internal Reports

### 2009-2013

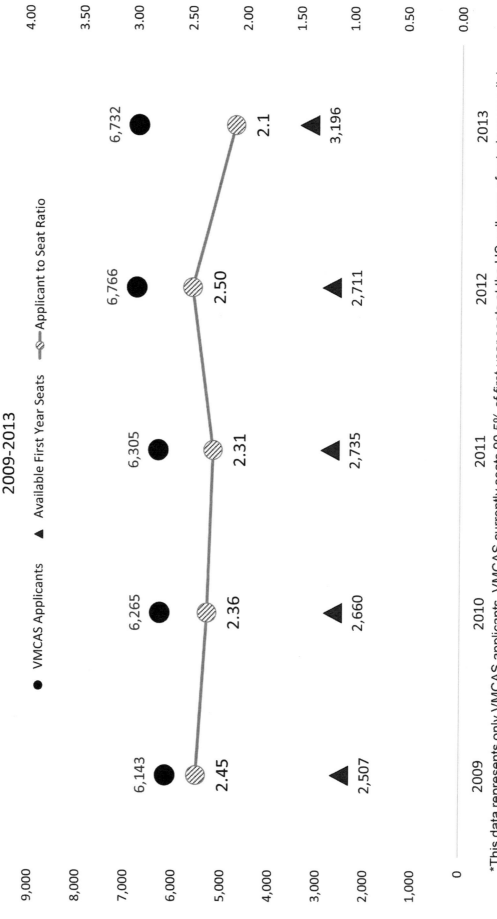

● VMCAS Applicants    ▲ Available First Year Seats    —⊘— Applicant to Seat Ratio

| | 2009 | 2010 | 2011 | 2012 | 2013 |
|---|---|---|---|---|---|
| VMCAS Applicants | 6,143 | 6,265 | 6,305 | 6,766 | 6,732 |
| Applicant to Seat Ratio | 2.45 | 2.36 | 2.31 | 2.50 | 2.1 |
| Available First Year Seats | 2,507 | 2,660 | 2,735 | 2,711 | 3,196 |

*This data represents only VMCAS applicants. VMCAS currently seats 90.5% of first-year seats at the US colleges of veterinary medicine. The fall 2014 (class of 2018) ratio is projected; it includes first-year seats created by the recent additions of Colleges of Veterinary Medicine at Midwestern University and Lincoln Memorial University. This data includes available seats at all VMCAS participating institutions, including non-US colleges of veterinary medicine.

171